HEALTH CARE IN TRANSITION

MEDICAID SPENDING BY STATES

VARIATIONS AND INFLUENCES

HEALTH CARE IN TRANSITION

Additional books in this series can be found on Nova's website under the Series tab.

Additional e-books in this series can be found on Nova's website under the e-book tab.

HEALTH CARE IN TRANSITION

MEDICAID SPENDING BY STATES

VARIATIONS AND INFLUENCES

HANK MILFORD
EDITOR

nova publishers
New York

For permission to use material from this book please contact us:
Telephone 631-231-7269; Fax 631-231-8175
Web Site: http://www.novapublishers.com

Additional color graphics may be available in the e-book version of this book.

Library of Congress Cataloging-in-Publication Data

ISBN: 978-1-63463-538-7

Published by Nova Science Publishers, Inc. † New York

CONTENTS

PREFACE

Medicaid is a means-tested entitlement program that finances the delivery of primary and acute medical services as well as long-term care. Medicaid is jointly funded by the federal government and the states. The federal government's share of a state's expenditures is called the federal medical assistance percentage (FMAP) rate. The remainder is referred to as the nonfederal share, or state share. Estimates of Medicaid spending developed from Centers for Medicare & Medicaid Services (CMS) data sources suggest wide variation among states in Medicaid spending per enrollee, overall and for each of four main eligibility groups—children, adults, disabled, and aged. This book examines Medicaid spending per enrollee by state; selected factors that influence Medicaid spending per enrollee, by state; and how states account for factors that influence expected per-enrollee spending when setting rates for Medicaid managed care plans.

Chapter 1 – Federal Medicaid expenditures totaled about $267 billion in fiscal year 2013. With the expansion of Medicaid under the Patient Protection and Affordable Care Act and rising health care costs, the Congressional Budget Office projects that such expenditures will grow to about $576 billion by fiscal year 2024. GAO was asked to examine variation among states in Medicaid spending and factors that influence such spending, and state approaches to setting rates per enrollee for Medicaid managed care plans.

This report examines (1) Medicaid spending per enrollee by state; (2) selected factors that influence Medicaid spending per enrollee, by state; and (3) how states account for factors that influence expected per-enrollee spending when setting rates for Medicaid managed care plans. GAO analyzed Medicaid enrollment and combined federal and state expenditure data provided by CMS for fiscal year 2008, and examined illustrative examples of factors that have been reported to influence health care spending, such as age, disability status, and scope of benefits received. GAO used 2008 data because they allowed a comparable view of spending per enrollee and factors that influence spending per enrollee—as 2008 was the most recent year for which certain data on factors influencing spending were readily available. GAO also interviewed officials in three states and five consulting firms with experience setting Medicaid managed care rates.

The Department of Health and Human Services provided technical comments on a draft of this report, which GAO incorporated as appropriate.

Chapter 2 – Medicaid is a means-tested entitlement program that finances the delivery of primary and acute medical services as well as long-term services and supports. Medicaid is a federal and state partnership that is jointly financed by both the federal government and the states.

The federal government's share for most Medicaid expenditures is called the federal medical assistance percentage (FMAP) rate. Generally determined annually, the FMAP formula is designed so that the federal government pays a larger portion of Medicaid costs in states with lower per capita incomes relative to the national average (and vice versa for states with higher per capita incomes). Federal Medicaid funding to states is open-ended.

The federal government provides states a good deal of flexibility in determining the composition of the state share (also referred to as the non-federal share) of Medicaid expenditures. As a result, there is significant variation from state to state in the funding sources used to finance the state share of Medicaid expenditures. In state FY2012, states reported that on average state general funds (i.e., revenues from personal income, sales, and corporate income taxes) made up 77% of the state share of Medicaid expenditures and the remaining 23% was financed by "other state funds" (i.e., provider taxes, local government funds, and tobacco settlement funds).

In FY2012, Medicaid expenditures totaled $431 billion, with the federal government paying $249 billion, about 58% of the total. While Medicaid expenditures (like all health expenditures) generally grow at a rate faster than the economy, as measured by the gross domestic product (GDP), spending per enrollee under Medicaid tends to be lower than the per person spending for other forms of health insurance. One of the major factors impacting Medicaid spending is the economy. Also, state-specific factors, such as programmatic decisions and demographics, affect Medicaid expenditures and cause Medicaid spending to vary widely from state to state.

Starting in FY2014, Medicaid expenditures are expected to increase significantly as a result of the reforms enacted in the Patient Protection and

Affordable Care Act (ACA, P.L. 111-148 as amended). The most noteworthy ACA change to Medicaid started January 1, 2014, when some states expanded Medicaid eligibility to adults under age 65 with income up to 133% of the federal poverty level (FPL) (effectively 138% FPL with the 5% FPL income disregard).

Following the June 28, 2012, Supreme Court decision in *National Federation of Independent Business v. Sebelius*, it is uncertain how many states will expand their Medicaid program to cover this new group. According to the Congressional Budget Office and the Joint Committee on Taxation, the expansion is expected to increase federal Medicaid expenditures by $612 billion from FY2014 to FY2022, which is $319 billion less than the estimate conducted prior to the Supreme Court decision.

This report provides an overview of Medicaid's financing structure, including both federal and state financing issues. The Medicaid expenditures section of the report discusses economic factors affecting Medicaid, state variability in spending, and projected program spending. Other issues that are examined include federal deficit reduction proposals affecting Medicaid and state fiscal conditions affecting Medicaid financing and services.

Chapter 3 – Medicaid is a means-tested entitlement program that finances the delivery of primary and acute medical services as well as long-term care. Medicaid is jointly funded by the federal government and the states. The federal government's share of a state's expenditures is called the federal medical assistance percentage (FMAP) rate. The remainder is referred to as the nonfederal share, or state share.

Generally determined annually, the FMAP formula is designed so that the federal government pays a larger portion of Medicaid costs in states with lower per capita incomes relative to the national average (and vice versa for states with higher per capita incomes). FMAP rates have a statutory minimum of 50% and a statutory maximum of 83%. For FY2014, regular FMAP rates range from 50.00% to 73.05%. The FMAP rate is used to reimburse states for the federal share of most Medicaid expenditures, but exceptions to the regular FMAP rate have been made for certain states, situations, populations, providers, and services.

Some recent issues related to FMAP include FMAP changes in the Patient Protection and Affordable Care Act (ACA, P.L. 111-148 as amended), federal deficit reduction proposals that would amend the FMAP rate, and the disaster-related FMAP adjustment.

The ACA contains a number of provisions affecting FMAP rates. Most notably, the ACA provides initial FMAP rates of up to 100% for certain "newly eligible" individuals. Also, under the ACA, "expansion states" receive an enhanced FMAP rate for certain individuals. In addition, ACA provides increased FMAP rates for certain disaster-affected states, primary care payment rate increases, specified preventive services and immunizations, smoking cessation services for pregnant women, specified home and community-based services, health home services for certain people with chronic conditions, home and community-based attendant services and supports, and state balancing incentive payments.

Since federal Medicaid expenditures are a large and growing portion of the federal budget, controlling federal Medicaid spending has been included in some federal deficit reduction proposals. Some of the federal deficit reduction proposals include provisions that would amend the current FMAP structure through either a blended FMAP or a reduction to the statutory FMAP floor.

The ACA included a provision providing a disaster-recovery FMAP adjustment for states that have experienced a major, statewide disaster. Louisiana is the only state that has been eligible for the disaster-recovery adjusted FMAP since the fourth quarter of FY2011 (when the adjustment was first available). Both the Middle Class Tax Relief and Job Creation Act of 2012 (P.L. 112-96) and the Moving Ahead for Progress in the 21st Century Act (MAP-21, P.L. 112-141) amended the formula for the disaster-recovery adjusted FMAP.

This report describes the FMAP calculation used to reimburse states for most Medicaid expenditures, and it lists the statutory exceptions to the regular FMAP rate. In addition, this report discusses other FMAP-related issues, including FMAP changes in ACA, federal deficit reduction proposals affecting the FMAP rate, and the disaster-recovery FMAP adjustment.

In: Medicaid Spending by States
Editor: Hank Milford
ISBN: 978-1-63463-538-7

Chapter 1

MEDICAID: ASSESSMENT OF VARIATION AMONG STATES IN PER-ENROLLEE SPENDING*

United States Government Accountability Office

WHY GAO DID THIS STUDY

Federal Medicaid expenditures totaled about $267 billion in fiscal year 2013. With the expansion of Medicaid under the Patient Protection and Affordable Care Act and rising health care costs, the Congressional Budget Office projects that such expenditures will grow to about $576 billion by fiscal year 2024. GAO was asked to examine variation among states in Medicaid spending and factors that influence such spending, and state approaches to setting rates per enrollee for Medicaid managed care plans.

This report examines (1) Medicaid spending per enrollee by state; (2) selected factors that influence Medicaid spending per enrollee, by state; and (3) how states account for factors that influence expected per-enrollee spending when setting rates for Medicaid managed care plans. GAO analyzed Medicaid enrollment and combined federal and state expenditure data provided by CMS for fiscal year 2008, and examined illustrative examples of factors that have been reported to influence health care spending, such as age,

* This is an edited, reformatted and augmented version of a United States Government Accountability Office publication, No. GAO-14-456, dated June 2014.

disability status, and scope of benefits received. GAO used 2008 data because they allowed a comparable view of spending per enrollee and factors that influence spending per enrollee—as 2008 was the most recent year for which certain data on factors influencing spending were readily available. GAO also interviewed officials in three states and five consulting firms with experience setting Medicaid managed care rates.

The Department of Health and Human Services provided technical comments on a draft of this report, which GAO incorporated as appropriate.

What GAO Found

Estimates of Medicaid spending developed from Centers for Medicare & Medicaid Services (CMS) data sources suggest wide variation among states in Medicaid spending per enrollee, overall and for each of four main eligibility groups—children, adults, disabled, and aged.

Although estimates of spending per enrollee are based on the best data readily available from CMS, these data do not permit full assessment of state spending variation. Limitations include the difficulty of determining spending on services enrollees received during a particular time period and lack of complete, accurate information about supplemental payments. GAO has previously recommended that CMS take steps to improve states' reporting of supplemental payments and that Congress consider requiring CMS to take such steps.

Certain factors that influence overall per-enrollee Medicaid spending, such as distribution of enrollees among eligibility groups, enrollee health service needs, and scope of benefits offered, varied widely by state. For example, in calendar year 2008, the percentage of enrollees in higher-need eligibility groups— individuals who are disabled or aged—ranged from about 15 percent to 38 percent across states.

States consider a range of demographic and health factors to predict expected spending per enrollee when setting Medicaid managed care rates. According to consulting firm officials, states often consider detailed information on enrollee heath status, particularly for aged and disabled enrollees.

ABBREVIATIONS

CDC	Centers for Disease Control and Prevention
CMS	Centers for Medicare & Medicaid Services
DSH	Disproportionate Share Hospital
FFS	fee-for-service
FMAP	Federal Medical Assistance Percentage
HHS	Department of Health and Human Services
MACPAC	Medicaid and CHIP Payment and Access Commission
MAX	Medicaid Analytic eXtract
MSIS	Medicaid Statistical Information System
OACT	Office of the Actuary
PCI	per capita income
PPACA	Patient Protection and Affordable Care Act
T-MSIS	Transformed-MSIS

* * *

June 16, 2014

The Honorable Orrin G. Hatch
Ranking Member
Committee on Finance
United States Senate

The Honorable Fred Upton
Chairman
Committee on Energy and Commerce
House of Representatives

In fiscal year 2013, Medicaid, the federal-state health coverage program for certain low-income individuals, had over 70 million enrollees and expenditures totaling about $460 billion.[1] Of these expenditures, the federal government financed about $267 billion, with the rest financed by the states. With the expansion of Medicaid under the Patient Protection and Affordable Care Act (PPACA) and rising health care costs, increased Medicaid enrollment and spending are expected over the next 10 years— with federal Medicaid expenditures projected to grow to about $576 billion by 2024.[2] Prior studies have shown considerable differences among states both in total

Medicaid spending and in average spending per enrollee. Much of the state variation in total Medicaid spending can be attributed to differences in enrollment, but the reasons for variation in average spending per enrollee are not as well understood.

States and the federal government are interested in better understanding and controlling Medicaid program spending. At the state level, this interest is reflected in payment reform proposals and strategies such as the use of managed care service delivery systems, in which states seek to control costs by contracting with health plans to cover services provided to Medicaid enrollees for a fixed, or capitated, monthly rate per enrollee.[3] At the federal level, Medicaid has been the focus of proposals to reform the structure of Medicaid financing and change the methods used to allocate funds across states. Some of these proposals would limit the amount of federal funding states receive, while other proposals aim to control spending by reducing the variation in average state spending per enrollee.[4]

As we have emphasized in prior work, to help ensure that Medicaid funds are allocated equitably, any new approach to program financing must take into account that the costs of providing Medicaid services can differ across states, due to a variety of factors.[5] These factors include the size of the Medicaid population and certain factors that influence states' costs of providing Medicaid services per enrollee, such as differences in the health service needs of enrollees and the cost of delivering health care. Such considerations have some parallels to how states set managed care capitation rates to take into account that the costs of providing Medicaid services can differ among plans depending on the health service needs and other characteristics of individuals enrolled in each plan.

Given concerns regarding Medicaid spending and the interest in program financing reform, you asked us to examine the variation among states in Medicaid spending and factors that influence state spending on Medicaid services for enrollees. In addition, because states have experience examining the factors that affect per-enrollee Medicaid spending in order to set capitation rates for health plans in their managed care programs, you asked us to examine states' approaches to setting these rates. In this report, we (1) examine what Centers for Medicare & Medicaid Services (CMS) data show about the variation among states in Medicaid spending per enrollee; (2) describe the variation among states in factors that influence Medicaid spending per enrollee; and (3) describe how states set capitation rates for Medicaid managed care plans to account for factors that influence plans' expected spending per enrollee.

To examine what CMS data show about the variation among states in Medicaid spending per enrollee, we developed estimates for federal fiscal year 2008 using Medicaid enrollment data and combined federal and state expenditure data provided by the CMS Office of the Actuary (OACT).[6] We chose fiscal year 2008 so that our estimates of Medicaid spending per enrollee were for the same year as the most readily available data on certain factors that influence this spending. We obtained from OACT (1) Medicaid enrollment data showing the number of full-yearequivalent enrollees, by state and eligibility group, which OACT calculated from enrollment data in the Medicaid Statistical Information System (MSIS),[7] and (2) Medicaid expenditure estimates broken out by state, eligibility group, and service type, which OACT estimated using enrollment and expenditure data from MSIS and expenditure data from the CMS-64 data system. Our estimates of per-enrollee spending based on these data include supplemental payments to providers that are not linked to individual enrollees, including Disproportionate Share Hospital (DSH) payments, but do not include administrative costs.[8] In our estimates of per-enrollee spending, we distributed DSH payments among eligibility groups based on each group's share of state spending for services provided in the types of facilities eligible to receive DSH payments. We also explored an alternative method of distributing DSH payments among eligibility groups. (See appendix I for more information about the methodology used by OACT to generate its estimates and our use of the OACT estimates to develop estimates of spending per enrollee.) To assess the reliability of the data, we reviewed documentation for these data sources, interviewed CMS officials knowledgeable about the data, and compared our estimates to those from other data sources. On the basis of this assessment, we excluded states with significant errors or omissions in fiscal year 2008 data from certain analyses.[9] We determined that for the rest of the states, the data were sufficiently reliable for our purposes.

To describe the variation among states in factors that influence Medicaid spending per enrollee, we analyzed differences among states on selected indicators of enrollee health service needs and the geographic costs of delivering health care services. We focused on indicators that have been reported to influence health care spending and were readily available from previously published sources of Medicaid data and other federal data, such as U.S. Census Bureau or Centers for Disease Control and Prevention (CDC) data. For indicators drawn from Medicaid data, we relied to the extent possible on the *Medicaid Analytic eXtract (MAX) 2008 Chartbook*, the most recent year available. [10] For certain Medicaid indicators that were not published in the

MAX 2008 Chartbook, we obtained data directly from the MSIS 2008 Annual Person Summary File and the MSIS 2008 State Summary DataMart.[11] We focused our review on 2008 fiscal or calendar year data for greater comparability with the readily available MAX data. We did not attempt to identify causal links between state Medicaid spending and factors that influence spending, nor did we analyze all factors that may influence such spending. To assess the reliability of the data, we reviewed documentation for these data sources and interviewed CMS officials knowledgeable about the data. On the basis of this assessment, we excluded four states—Arizona, New Mexico, Wisconsin, and Maine—from analyses related to long-term care service use.[12] We excluded one state—Massachusetts—from all analyses based on the MSIS 2008 Annual Person Summary File or MSIS 2008 State Summary DataMart.[13] Otherwise, we determined that the data were sufficiently reliable for our purposes.

To describe how states set Medicaid managed care capitation rates to account for factors that influence plans' expected spending per enrollee, we reviewed documents from consulting firms, states, and CMS, as well as information from other sources, regarding how states establish Medicaid managed care capitation rates. We also interviewed officials at five consulting firms that have worked with at least 40 states to establish state Medicaid managed care capitation rates.[14] In addition, we interviewed officials from three states regarding their experiences establishing such capitation rates,[15] and interviewed CMS officials about the managed care data that CMS receives from states. Our review focused on how states account for factors influencing Medicaid spending, and we did not examine other aspects of the rate setting process, such as documenting the actuarial soundness of rates.

We conducted this performance audit from February 2013 to June 2014 in accordance with generally accepted government auditing standards. Those standards require that we plan and perform the audit to obtain sufficient, appropriate evidence to provide a reasonable basis for our findings and conclusions based on our audit objectives. We believe that the evidence obtained provides a reasonable basis for our findings and conclusions based on our audit objectives.

BACKGROUND

Each state administers its Medicaid program in accordance with its own Medicaid plan—which must be reviewed and approved by CMS—and determines, among other things, the groups of individuals covered, services provided, and the service delivery system, such as fee-forservice (FFS) or managed care. Within broad federal requirements, states have flexibility in deciding which individuals to cover and the range of medical services to provide in their Medicaid programs. For example, states must cover certain groups of individuals, such as children and pregnant women, but may elect to cover these groups above the required minimum income levels. States' Medicaid programs generally must cover a set of mandatory services, including those provided by primary and specialty care physicians, as well as services provided in hospitals, clinics, and other settings. States may also elect to cover additional optional benefits and services, such as home- and community-based services or rehabilitative services.[16] Subject to federal requirements, states have discretion in establishing the amount, duration, and scope of the mandatory and optional services covered in their Medicaid programs and may place appropriate limits on services based on certain criteria; thus, states may limit the number of visits or the days of care that are provided. In some cases, not all Medicaid enrollees are eligible for all covered services, such as those who receive only family planning benefits through demonstration waivers, or those who only qualify to receive assistance with Medicare premiums and cost sharing.[17]

States and the federal government share in the financing of the Medicaid program, with the federal government matching most state expenditures for Medicaid services on the basis of a statutory formula known as the Federal Medical Assistance Percentage (FMAP).[18] States pay health care providers or managed care plans for covered services provided to Medicaid enrollees, and then submit claims to CMS in order to receive federal matching funds for these payments. In addition to payments made directly to providers or managed care plans for services provided to enrollees, most states receive federal matching funds for other types of Medicaid payments, known as supplemental payments. For example, federal Medicaid law requires states to make DSH payments to qualifying hospitals that serve large numbers of Medicaid and uninsured low-income patients. States are required to report to CMS separate data on the two types of DSH payments: payments to inpatient hospitals and payments to inpatient mental health facilities.[19] States also make other supplemental payments, which we refer to as non-DSH supplemental payments, to hospitals and other providers that, for example, serve high-cost Medicaid enrollees.[20] Unlike regular Medicaid payments, supplemental payments are not necessarily made on the basis of claims for specific services to individual enrollees.

CMS maintains two readily available sources of data on state Medicaid spending: the CMS-64 data set and MSIS. [21] MSIS also contains state enrollment data. These two data sources have different roles and structures, and taken together have the potential to provide a robust picture of Medicaid spending.

- The CMS-64 data set contains aggregate state data on program-benefit and administrative spending by quarter, such as each state's total quarterly expenditures for inpatient hospital services or prescription drugs. The CMS-64 data set also contains information on spending not linked to specific enrollees, such as DSH and other supplemental payments, but no information on spending for individual enrollees or on the services they received under Medicaid.[22] States submit the CMS-64 quarterly data in order to obtain reimbursement for the federal share of Medicaid expenditures. CMS reviews the CMS-64 submissions, and the data are the most reliable accounting of total Medicaid spending available. However, because the CMS-64 does not include enrollee-specific data it cannot be used on its own to assess per-enrollee spending. The CMS-64 data system is programmed to produce two reports that summarize states' total spending for a given fiscal year; the reports differ primarily in their treatment of states' subsequent adjustments to their reported spending.
- MSIS is a national enrollment and claims data set and the federal source of Medicaid spending data that can be linked to specific enrollees on the basis of their medical claims for care.[23] Unlike the CMS-64 data set, however, MSIS only contains information about Medicaid expenditures that are tied to specific enrollees, and thus does not include some provider payments such as DSH or non-DSH supplemental payments. Although CMS reviews these data for reliability and uses them for policy analysis, program utilization, and forecasting spending, it does not use these data to determine the federal share of states' Medicaid expenditures, nor do states use the data to manage the daily operations of their Medicaid programs. CMS is in the process of implementing a project to improve and expand MSIS, but the time frames for completion are uncertain.[24]

Estimates of per-enrollee Medicaid spending can be obtained by combining the more reliable aggregated spending data from the CMS-64 with detailed enrollee-level information available from MSIS. For example, estimates of overall Medicaid spending per enrollee for a given fiscal year can be obtained by dividing total Medicaid expenditures, as shown in the annual state summary reports available from the CMS-64 data system, by total state Medicaid enrollment as derived from MSIS. In addition, through a more complex process, estimates of per-enrollee spending can be developed for particular eligibility groups. For example, the CMS-64 expenditures can be distributed among the four major Medicaid eligibility groups—children, adults, disabled, and aged—based on MSIS expenditure patterns by eligibility group.[25]

CMS Data Suggest Wide Variation among States in Medicaid Spending per Enrollee, but Data Limitations Hinder a More Complete Assessment

Estimates of Medicaid spending per enrollee developed from CMS data sources suggest wide variation among states. However, due to certain data limitations, these estimates do not permit full assessment of differences in per-enrollee spending among states.

CMS Data Suggest Wide Variation in Spending per Enrollee

CMS data suggest wide variation among states in Medicaid spending per enrollee, both overall and for each of the four major Medicaid eligibility groups—children, adults, disabled, and aged. Estimates based on expenditure data from CMS-64 annual summary reports and enrollment and expenditure data from MSIS indicate that overall spending per enrollee ranged from about $3,800 in California to about $11,700 in Rhode Island in fiscal year 2008.[26] (See fig. 1 for a general comparison of per-enrollee spending levels across states, and table 1 in appendix II for specific state-by-state estimates.)

These data also suggest wide variation among states in spending per enrollee by eligibility group. (See fig. 2.) For example, estimated per-enrollee spending for disabled enrollees ranged from about $9,000 in Alabama to over $32,000 in New York; and per-enrollee spending for aged enrollees ranged from about $10,000 to about $30,000 for these two states. (See table 1 in appendix II for state-by-state estimates.) The variation in estimated per-enrollee spending was smaller for the adult and child eligibility groups than for the disabled and aged groups, but was still substantial. For example, in fiscal year 2008, the estimates indicate that Vermont spent more than three times as much per child and per adult as California (about $5,900 versus about $1,700 for children, and about $5,700 versus about $1,500 for adults).

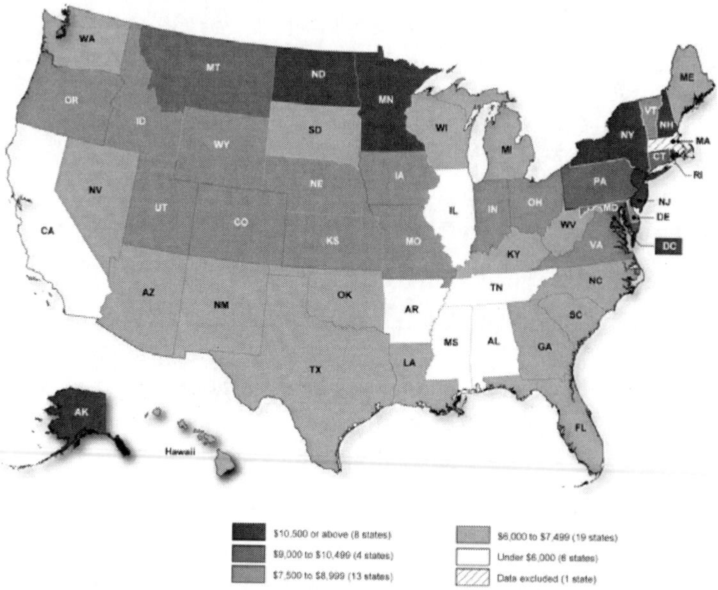

Source: GAO analysis of Centers for Medicare & Medicaid Services data; Map Resources (map). | GAO-14-456.

Notes: Estimates of spending per enrollee include federal and state spending on regular Medicaid payments to providers and managed care plans for covered services provided to enrollees, as well as Disproportionate Share Hospital (DSH) and non-DSH supplemental payments, but do not include administrative costs. Estimates also do not reflect states' subsequent changes, including adjustments or collections, to the spending originally reported for this year. Enrollment is measured in terms of fullyear-equivalent enrollees. Both enrollment and expenditure data include all enrollees, regardless of the scope of benefits offered. For purposes of this analysis, we include the District of Columbia as a state. We excluded Massachusetts because of errors in fiscal year 2008 CMS data for this state.

Figure 1. Estimated Medicaid Spending per Enrollee, by State, Fiscal Year 2008.

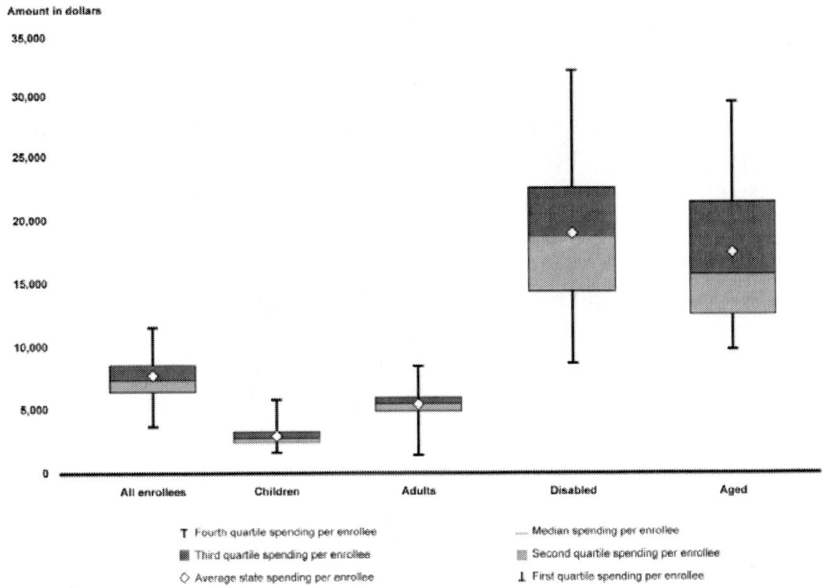

Source: GAO analysis of Centers for Medicare & Medicaid Services data. | GAO-14-456.

Notes: Spending per enrollee includes federal and state spending on regular Medicaid payments to providers and managed care plans for covered services provided to enrollees as well as Disproportionate Share Hospital (DSH) and non-DSH supplemental payments, but does not include administrative costs. Estimates also do not reflect states' subsequent changes, including adjustments or collections, to the spending originally reported for this year. Enrollment is measured in terms of fullyear-equivalent enrollees. Both enrollment and expenditure data include all enrollees, regardless of the scope of benefits offered. We excluded Massachusetts from all calculations and Maine from calculations at the eligibility group level because of errors or omissions in fiscal year 2008 data for these states. Average state spending per enrollee represents the sum of each state's spending per enrollee divided by the number of states. For purposes of this analysis, we include the District of Columbia as a state. Each box in the figure denotes the dollar range for states in the second and third quartiles in spending per enrollee. The horizontal line between the boxes denotes the median, the diamond denotes the average, and the vertical lines extending above and below each box denote the highest and lowest quartile state spending per enrollee.

Figure 2. Estimated State Medicaid Spending per Enrollee, by Eligibility Group, Fiscal Year 2008.

Data Limitations Hinder Assessment of State Variation in Spending per Enrollee

Although these estimates of spending per enrollee are based on the best data readily available from CMS Medicaid data sets—expenditure data from annual summary reports from the CMS-64 data set and expenditure and enrollment data from MSIS—they do not permit a full assessment of variation in per-enrollee spending among states, due to certain limitations of the CMS-64 data. These limitations include (1) the difficulty of determining spending on services received by enrollees during a specific time period, and (2) the lack of complete, accurate information about supplemental payments. These limitations constrain the accuracy of per-enrollee spending estimates based on these data, particularly at the eligibility group level, and thus hinder a complete assessment of how spending varies among states.

Difficulty of Determining Spending on Services Received during a Specific Time Period

The first data limitation is that annual summary reports currently available from the CMS-64 data system do not accurately reflect spending on the services that were provided to enrollees during the year. This is because, in these annual reports, the spending originally reported for the year is not updated to account for adjustments to that spending, or collections, that states report in subsequent years.[27] For example, if a state reports spending $500 million for nursing facility care in a given year, but then adjusts that amount up by $50 million, it is not possible to ascertain from the annual reports that the state's actual spending for this care in this year was $550 million.

While these reports provide accurate records of the amount of expenditures states reported to CMS in a fiscal year to claim their federal matching funds—the programmatic purpose for which they were designed—the treatment of adjustments and collections in these reports limits the accuracy of estimates of per-enrollee spending based on these data. For example, in one of the two summary reports that provide data on states' total spending by type of service, all adjustments reported by a state that year are summed by type—for example, adjustments increasing claims—and reported as separate line items.[28] The reported sums may include adjustments applicable to spending for the current year as well as prior years.[29] As a result, neither including nor excluding the adjustments in the total spending shown in the report for a given year will yield an accurate picture of states' spending on the services provided to enrollees that year.[30] Collections received by the states that apply to previous year claims are also reported as a line item in the summary reports for the year in which they were reported rather than the year of the claims to which they apply.[31]

Because the amount of adjustments and collections relative to current year spending is not consistent across states and fluctuates over time in some states, estimates of per-enrollee spending based on these annual summary reports, in combination with MSIS data, are not comparable across states or over time. The large amount of adjustments and collections reported by some states in fiscal year 2008 suggests that the states' actual spending for the services received by enrollees that year could differ significantly from estimates that do not account for these changes. For example, adjustments and collections represented 24 percent of reported spending for California in fiscal year 2008 and 5 to 9 percent of reported spending for five other states.[32] (See table 2 in appendix III for state-by-state data on total spending and adjustments and collections.)

The effect of the adjustments and collections may be magnified when per-enrollee spending is estimated separately by eligibility group. To the extent that certain eligibility groups account for a disproportionate share of the spending that a state subsequently adjusts, failure to apply those adjustments to the original spending will disproportionately affect estimates of the spending for services provided to that group of enrollees. For example, because aged or disabled enrollees account for a greater share of spending for institutional long-term care, an adjustment to spending for that care will affect estimates of spending for aged or disabled enrollees more than those for children or adults.

While the CMS-64 annual summary reports do not apply adjustments or collections to spending for the relevant time periods, the information needed to apply most of these changes is available in the CMS-64 data system. In fiscal year 2008, adjustments accounted for most of the changes states reported to their spending—particularly in states where adjustments and collections were highest relative to total spending—and states are required to report not only the dollar amount of adjustments, but also the time period to which they apply.[33] (For collections, states are required to report only the dollar amount.) Although this detailed information about adjustments is available in the CMS-64 data system, CMS officials told us that the system has not been programmed to produce a report that updates reported spending to account for subsequent adjustments. To manually extract and compile this information in order to apply adjustments to the correct time period of spending would be a laborious process that could involve compiling information from dozens of reports.[34]

Lack of Complete, Accurate Information about Supplemental Payments

The second data limitation is the lack of complete and accurate information about states' use of supplemental payments, and the consequent uncertainty about whether and how these payments should be included in estimates of Medicaid spending per enrollee, particularly at the eligibility group level. This information gap is partly due to historical differences in the reporting requirements for the two types of supplemental payments: DSH and non-DSH. CMS requires states to report DSH payments as a separate line item in their CMS-64 reports, but the agency did not require states to separately report non-DSH supplemental payments until fiscal year 2010. [35] As we have previously reported, state reporting of non-DSH payments in the CMS-64 was incomplete in 2010,[36] and according to CMS officials, reporting is still incomplete, as some states continue to fold at least some non-DSH supplemental payments into the spending reported for related services.[37] As a result, it is not possible to exclude non-DSH supplemental payments from the spending reported in the CMS-64 prior to fiscal year 2010, or to fully exclude these payments from the spending reported in the following years. Since some states appear to use non-DSH supplemental payments more than DSH payments, while others appear to do the reverse,[38] excluding one type of supplemental payment from estimates of per-enrollee spending while including another would skew comparisons among states. For this reason, we included DSH payments in our estimates of per-enrollee spending.

Even if it were possible to exclude both types of payments from estimates of per-enrollee spending, it is not clear that it would be appropriate to do so. Some researchers have suggested that supplemental payments should not be included, or should not be included in their entirety, in estimates of spending for Medicaid enrollees because these funds are intended to offset providers' uncompensated care costs not only for Medicaid enrollees but also for uninsured low- income individuals. 39 However, it could also be argued that these payments should be included in estimates of per-enrollee spending because it is possible that states' use of these payments may relate to how much they pay providers directly for the services furnished to enrollees. For example, if hospitals have higher uncompensated care costs in states with lower base payment rates, this would make these facilities eligible for larger DSH payments.

Including supplemental payments in estimates of spending per enrollee by eligibility group requires judgment as to the share of payments that should be attributed to each group. For fiscal year 2008, this judgment concerns only DSH payments, as non-DSH supplemental payments were folded into payments for services rather than separately reported. Our analysis found that how DSH payments are distributed among eligibility groups can significantly affect estimates of spending per enrollee by eligibility group, particularly for states with relatively high DSH payments.[40] We examined two possible distribution methods, each of which has advantages and disadvantages.

- One possible method is to distribute DSH payments among eligibility groups based on each group's share of spending for relevant services—for example, to distribute inpatient hospital DSH payments based on states' reported spending for services provided in these facilities (hospital inpatient and outpatient services).[41] This method is intended to assign to each eligibility group a share of DSH payments that reflects that group's relative use of services at the types of facilities that are potentially eligible for these payments. However, because states report spending on hospital inpatient and outpatient services only for enrollees who receive care on an FFS basis, this method may disproportionately assign inpatient DSH dollars to eligibility groups that are less likely to be enrolled in comprehensive managed care programs.[42] If, for example, none of a state's disabled and aged enrollees are in comprehensive managed care, while all of the state's child and adult enrollees are, the only FFS claims in MSIS for hospital inpatient and outpatient care would be for disabled and aged enrollees. Accordingly, under this method, all inpatient DSH funds would be assigned to these two eligibility groups, regardless of the amount of hospital inpatient and outpatient services children and adults received that were covered under managed care capitation payments.
- A second possible method is to distribute DSH payments among eligibility groups based on each group's share of total spending, including both FFS claims and capitation payments. This method takes into account spending for enrollees in managed care plans, but assigns DSH dollars to eligibility groups based partly on their spending for services that are not provided in facilities eligible for DSH payments. For example, the share of inpatient hospital DSH payments assigned to the aged eligibility group under this method would be based not only on their spending for inpatient and outpatient hospital services, but also on their spending for institutional long-term care, which constitutes a larger proportion of their overall spending.

For some eligibility groups in some states, the inclusion of DSH payments substantially increases estimates of spending per enrollee for fiscal year 2008. The amount of that increase varies depending on which of the two methods described above is used to distribute DSH payments. In three states, estimates of spending per enrollee for some groups differed by more than $1,000 depending on the distribution method used. For example, in New Hampshire—the state for which the choice of distribution method makes the greatest dollar difference—the difference in Medicaid spending per enrollee for adults in fiscal year 2008 was $2,123—$8,508 using the first method and $6,385 using the second method (see fig. 3, and see table 3 in app. IV for state-by-state estimates).

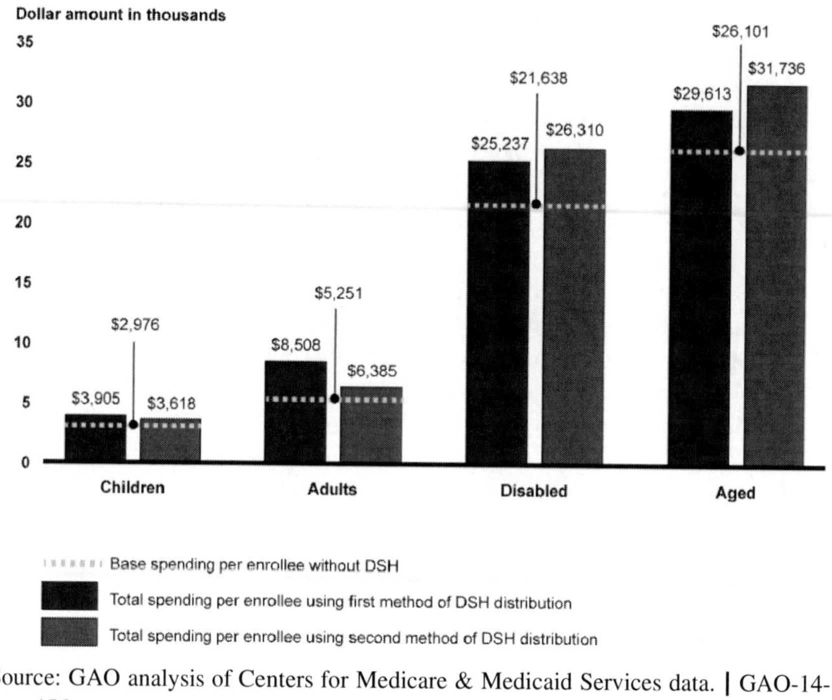

Source: GAO analysis of Centers for Medicare & Medicaid Services data. | GAO-14-456.

Notes: Spending per enrollee includes federal and state spending on regular Medicaid payments to providers and managed care plans for covered services provided to enrollees as well as DSH and non-DSH supplemental payments, but does not include administrative costs. Estimates also do not reflect states' subsequent changes, including adjustments or collections, to the spending originally reported for this year.

Enrollment is measured in terms of full-year-equivalent enrollees. Both enrollment and expenditure data include all enrollees regardless of the scope of benefits offered.

The first method distributes DSH payments among eligibility groups based on each group's share of spending for services delivered in the types of facilities that are potentially eligible for DSH payments. The second method distributes DSH payments among eligibility groups based on each group's share of total non-DSH spending.

Figure 3. Estimated Medicaid Spending per Enrollee in New Hampshire Using Two Possible Methods of Distributing Disproportionate Share Hospital (DSH) Payments, Fiscal Year 2008.

States Varied Widely on Program Characteristics and Other Factors That Influence Medicaid Per-Enrollee Spending

We found that the distribution of enrollees among the four major Medicaid eligibility groups (children, adults, disabled, and aged)—a program characteristic known to influence overall per-enrollee Medicaid spending—varied widely between states. Additionally, states varied on other selected factors that influence Medicaid spending for each of the four eligibility groups, including enrollee health services needs, scope of benefits offered, and the cost of delivering health services.

Distribution of Enrollees across Medicaid Eligibility Groups Varies by State

The distribution of enrollees across the disabled, aged, adult, and child eligibility groups varies widely by state. For example, the percentage of enrollees in the higher-need disabled and aged eligibility groups ranged from about 15 percent in Arizona to 38 percent in West Virginia in calendar year 2008.[43] (See fig. 4, and see table 5 in app. VI for full information on all states.)

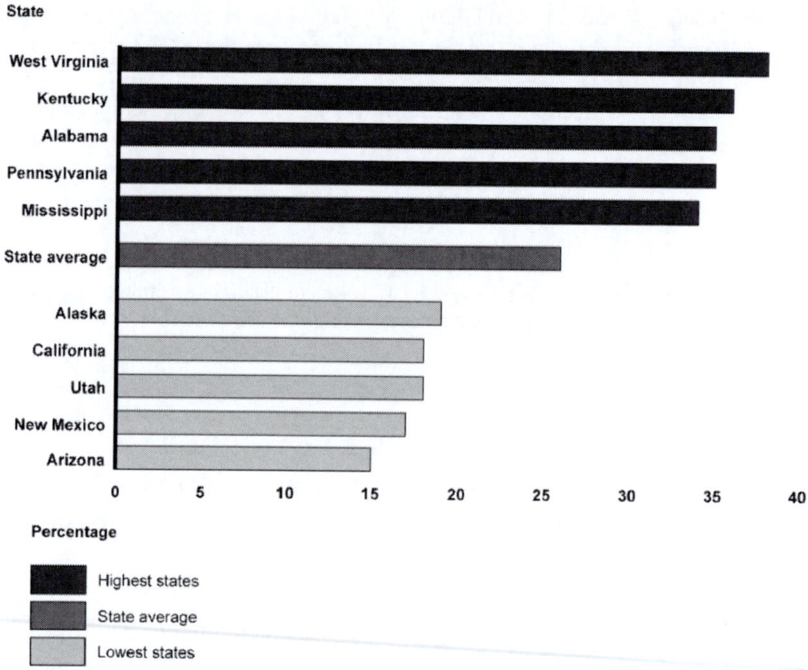

Source: GAO analysis of Centers for Medicare & Medicaid Services data. | GAO-14-456.

Notes: State average represents the sum of state percentages of enrollees who were disabled or aged divided by the number of states. For purposes of this analysis, we include the District of Columbia as a state.

Figure 4. Percentage of Medicaid Enrollees Who Were Disabled or Aged, Highest and Lowest Five States, Calendar Year 2008.

Differences across states in the distribution of Medicaid enrollees across eligibility groups occur due to multiple factors, such as the age distribution and rate of disability within each state's Medicaid-eligible population, as well as Medicaid eligibility rules. State-specific data on the characteristics of the population in poverty—a proxy for the Medicaid-eligible population—illustrate variation in age and disability rates. For example, calendar year 2008 U.S. Census Bureau American Community Survey data show that the percentage of the population in poverty who were aged 75 or older ranged from 1 percent in Alaska to 9 percent in North Dakota, while the percentage of the working-age population in poverty who reported a disability ranged from 17 percent in Utah to 39 percent in Maine. In addition, one state may have a higher percentage of aged or disabled Medicaid enrollees than another due to a variety of circumstances, such as having a higher income eligibility limit for aged or disabled individuals than another state, or conversely, having lower income eligibility limits for other groups.

Health Service Needs, Benefits, and Cost of Delivering Services Vary by State

Differences between states in the distribution of enrollees among the four major eligibility groups do not fully explain the variation among states in overall per-enrollee Medicaid spending, as states also vary in spending for each of the four eligibility groups. Although the Medicaid eligibility group itself is a key indicator of enrollees' average health service needs, the needs of individual enrollees within each group can differ substantially. As a result, the proportion of each Medicaid eligibility group that requires and uses higher-cost health services can vary by state. For example, the aged eligibility group includes a broad age range of individuals aged 65 and older. The chances of needing long-term care services, some of the most costly services covered by Medicaid, are higher for older enrollees within the aged eligibility group, and some states have a higher percentage of older enrollees than others. The proportion of enrollees in the aged eligibility group who were aged 85 and older ranged from 16.6 percent in Nevada to 38.9 percent in South Dakota in fiscal year 2008, according to our analysis of MSIS data. Across states with available data, the proportion of aged enrollees receiving long-term care services ranged from 18.4 percent in Florida to 65.6 percent in Iowa.[44] (See fig. 5, and see table 6 in app. VII for full information on all states.)

Furthermore, the proportion of enrollees in specific eligibility groups who received long-term care services in institutional settings, which are typically more costly than home- and community-based services, also varied among states.[45] Among states with available data, the proportion of aged enrollees who received institutional care ranged from 8.2 percent in Alaska to 46.1 percent in North Dakota.[46] (See table 6 in app. VII for full information on all states.) The setting in which long-term care services are provided may reflect factors other than or in addition to enrollees' health services needs, including state policy choices such as funding for home- and community-based services.

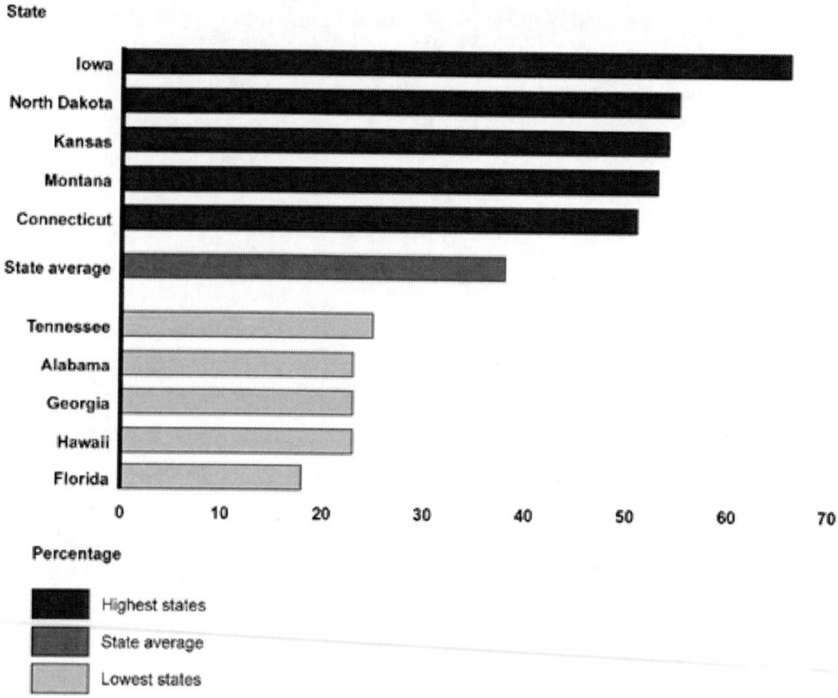

Source: GAO analysis of Centers for Medicare & Medicaid Services data. | GAO-14-456.

Notes: Four states were excluded because they did not have reliable data available on the proportion of aged enrollees receiving long-term care services. Specifically, in Arizona, New Mexico, and Wisconsin, more than 2 percent of all enrollees—and therefore likely a higher percentage of aged enrollees—received long-term care services through managed care plans and therefore were not represented in the fee-for-service data used to identify enrollees who received long-term care services during the year. Maine was unable to accurately report its spending by service category. A fifth state, Massachusetts, was excluded because of errors in fiscal year 2008 data. State average represents the sum of state percentages of aged enrollees receiving long-term care services divided by the number of states. For purposes of this analysis, we include the District of Columbia as a state.

Figure 5. Percentage of Aged Medicaid Enrollees Receiving Long-Term Care Services, Highest and Lowest Five States, Fiscal Year 2008.

The health service needs of Medicaid enrollees in the child and adult eligibility groups also vary by state. For example, research has documented that foster children have more health problems, especially mental health problems, than the general population or the population of poor children, and thus tend to generate higher health care spending. 47 Across states, the proportion of the child eligibility category that is composed of children enrolled in Medicaid on the basis of being in foster care ranged from about 1 percent in Mississippi to about 11 percent in Nebraska in fiscal year 2008, according to our analysis of MSIS data. Among adults, certain indicators of greater health service needs and costs, such as obesity and tobacco use, also vary by state.[48] Across states, calendar year 2008 CDC Behavioral Risk Factor Surveillance System data show that adult obesity rates ranged from 19 percent in Colorado to 33 percent in Mississippi, and tobacco use rates ranged from 10 percent in Utah to 26 percent in Kentucky and West Virginia. (See table 7 in app. VII for full information on all states.)

The scope of benefits offered to enrollees within the same eligibility group is another factor that influences Medicaid spending, and this also varies across states. Expenditures for enrollees with limited benefits are considerably lower than for those enrollees who are entitled to the full range of benefits offered by their state. For example, average per-enrollee spending was $205 for enrollees receiving only family planning services in calendar year 2008, compared with $5,281 for enrollees eligible for the full range of benefits offered in the state.[49] As a result, inclusion of spending data for enrollees with limited benefits, such as those receiving only family planning benefits, lowers a state's estimated average spending for an eligibility group as a whole. The proportion of enrollees with limited benefits can vary widely by state: the percentage of adult enrollees with only family planning benefits varied from 0 percent in 27 states to over 41 percent in 3 states in calendar year 2008.[50] (See fig. 6, and see table 7 in app. VII for full information on all states.)

The overall scope of benefits for enrollees receiving full benefits also varies by state. States may vary the amount, duration, or scope of benefits they are required to offer. States may also choose which, if any, optional benefits to offer. For example, dental services are an optional benefit for adults. State dental coverage for adults ranges from no coverage to full coverage. Dental services add to total per-enrollee spending for the adult eligibility group in states that cover such services for adults.

Another factor that influences state Medicaid spending per enrollee and varies across states is the cost of delivering health services to enrollees. The cost to states of delivering health services includes not only medical equipment and supplies, but also costs that vary considerably by location due to different labor market and real estate market factors. Of these, personnel costs represent the greatest proportion of total health service costs. In a previous report, we calculated the average 2009 through 2011 wages, by state, for health care workers, and used the differences between states in average wages to estimate how the costs of providing health care services varied by state.[51] The most conservatively calculated estimates showed an 18 percentage point difference between states in the cost of delivering health services.[52]

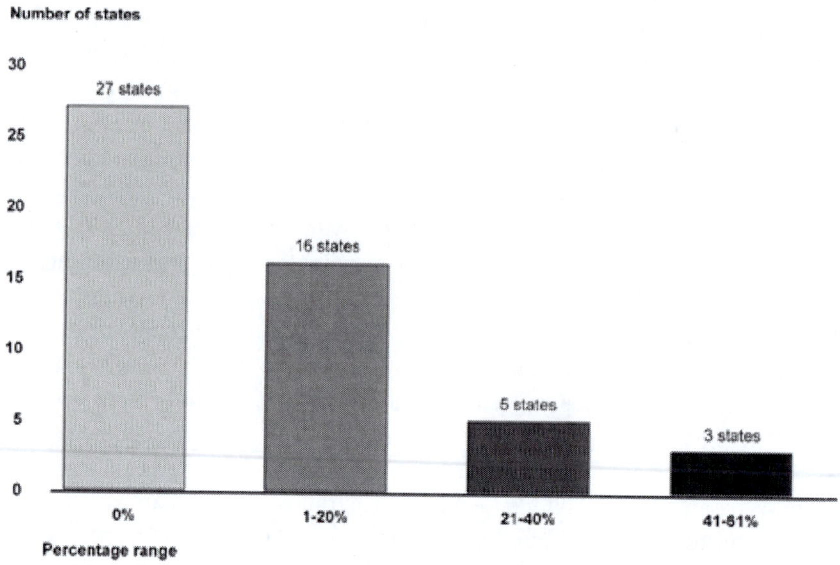

Source: GAO analysis of Centers for Medicare & Medicaid Services data. | GAO-14-456.

Note: For purposes of this analysis, we include the District of Columbia as a state.

Figure 6. Variation across States in the Percentage of Adult Medicaid Enrollees Who Received Only Family Planning Benefits, Calendar Year 2008.

States Account for a Range of Demographic and Health Factors When Setting Medicaid Managed Care Rates

States consider a range of factors when setting Medicaid managed care capitation rates to account for differences among plans in expected spending per enrollee. The number and complexity of factors considered varies based, in part, on the populations and benefits covered through managed care, as well as on state experience with managed care. States' considerations offer insight into the range of factors that influence per-enrollee spending at the state level and that contribute to the variation among states in such spending.

Officials from two consulting firms told us that some states are able to set sufficiently accurate rates—particularly for children and adults—by dividing enrollees into categories, known as rate cells. States pay distinct rates for enrollees in each cell based on the historical average spending for enrollees in the rate cell. The goal is for each rate cell to contain enrollees expected to generate relatively similar expenses; thus, states divide enrollees into rate cells based on eligibility and demographic data associated with health service needs and costs of delivering services, such as Medicaid eligibility group, age, gender, and geographic area. For example, states may divide children into multiple age group cells, and each of these rate cells may further differ depending on geographic area. The number of rate cells can vary widely across states. Officials from one consulting firm noted that states may use as few as 10 or more than 50 rate cells depending on their analysis of prior costs for enrollees in each cell.

Beyond demographic information, some states consider additional factors in establishing rate cells, such as receipt of high-cost services or the scope of benefits to which enrollees are entitled. For example, some state and consulting firm officials noted that states may establish separate rate cells for those with certain high-cost health needs, such as enrollees who are in neonatal intensive care, living with the human immunodeficiency virus or acquired immunodeficiency syndrome, dependent on ventilators, or in long-term care. Some states establish separate rate cells for children who are eligible for Medicaid on the basis of foster care, due to the greater health needs of foster children compared to other children.[53] In addition, states that offer different benefit packages to enrollees in specific eligibility groups may further divide such enrollees into distinct rate cells.

In addition to establishing rate cells, states that cover aged and disabled enrollees under managed care generally use risk adjustment to set rates based on detailed encounter data that provide information on enrollee health status, such as medical diagnoses or pharmacy prescriptions. 54 The risk adjustment process generally uses health status information, along with demographic factors, to predict the extent to which a particular enrollee is expected to require higher or lower spending than an average enrollee in the same rate cell. This information is used to proportionally adjust payments to managed care plans upward or downward. Specifically, plans enrolling a greater than average proportion of individuals who are expected to have costly health service needs receive proportionally higher payments, while plans enrolling a lower proportion of such individuals receive proportionally lower payments, and the state's overall payment remains unchanged. The types of health status data that can be incorporated in the risk adjustment process include diagnosed medical conditions, such as hypertension or asthma, along with other factors, such as age or gender. Some states also consider other types of health data in the risk adjustment process. For example, officials from one consulting firm told us that, for long-term care enrollees, some states are developing methods to incorporate assessments of frailty or ability to perform activities of daily living, such as the ability to walk or dress without assistance. Officials from two consulting firms told us that risk adjustment is particularly important for enrollees with the most variation in health service needs, such as disabled or aged enrollees, for whom age or other demographic factors are poor predictors of service use.

According to state and consulting firm officials, states that use risk adjustment tend to be those with more managed care experience, because these states (1) tend to use managed care to cover the disabled and aged eligibility groups whose health service needs vary more and for whom risk adjustment therefore is most important; and (2) are more likely to have made the data improvements necessary to use risk adjustment.[55] Risk adjustment requires detailed encounter data to measure health status;[56] however, some states do not have reliable and accurate encounter data.[57] Some of these officials said it has generally taken states about 3 to 4 years to transition to risk adjustment from rate setting based solely on rate cells, due to the need to educate providers and plans about appropriately reporting encounter data and due to other considerations, such as changes to information technology systems and the potential need to phase in rate changes.[58]

Despite states' use of multiple factors to predict health service needs for rate setting purposes, the need for certain services remains difficult to predict, and many states find it necessary to exclude such services from capitation rates—instead they may provide one-time payments for such services or exclude them from the package of services that managed care plans provide. For example, officials from several states and consulting firms mentioned that some states pay plans an additional fixed amount per enrollee to cover maternity-related services. Officials from two consulting firms also noted that some states use additional payments for enrollees who need certain high-cost services, such as organ transplants or neonatal intensive care. Alternately, states may exclude or "carve out" certain services or specific enrollee populations from coverage, rather than accounting for these costs in capitation rates. Officials from several states and consulting firms noted examples of services that some states exclude, such as maternity care or mental health, or enrollee populations that some states exclude, such as those receiving substance abuse treatment or children with special needs. States may use FFS or specific benefit plans, such as mental health or pharmacy plans, to cover these services or enrollees.

In the event that rates significantly differ from the actual average per-enrollee spending of managed care plans, states have also adopted various risk mitigation strategies to minimize the losses or gains that may be incurred by either the state or managed care plans. These strategies include

- *reinsurance*—requiring managed care plans to obtain private or state-financed insurance against unexpected expenses that may be significantly higher than the capitation rate payments they receive from the state, and
- *risk corridors*—limiting the losses or gains that states or managed care plans can incur, such as limiting the profits that a managed care plan could receive if capitation payments were significantly higher than plan spending.

Without these strategies, states risk paying more than necessary if capitation rates are too high, and managed care plans may not be willing to participate in a state's Medicaid program if rates are too low. Officials from one firm told us that rates based on poor data have resulted in states paying plans too much, or conversely, plans losing money on state Medicaid contracts.

Officials from one state and one consulting firm told us that states' reliance on risk mitigation strategies generally decreases as their managed care programs mature and the accuracy of their capitation rates increases. However, such strategies can continue to play an important role in the event of changes in circumstances, such as changes in the enrollee population due to economic conditions. For example, officials from one state with a long history of managed care experience told us that the state had considered dropping its risk corridors, but decided they still were necessary to limit managed care plan profits because the current adult Medicaid population—which increased during the recent recession—was healthier on average than the prior population on which rates were based.[59]

Concluding Observations

Understanding the variation among states in Medicaid spending is important for program oversight and for informing potential financing reform strategies. While the variation in overall spending among states is driven in large part by each state's Medicaid enrollment, it is also due to differences in spending per enrollee. The reasons for spending differences are not well understood, and some reasons for the differences may be within states' control—such as the extent to which states offer optional or limited benefits to enrollees. However, spending variation may also be due to different circumstances faced by states, such as geographic cost differences or the extent of enrollee health service needs, which are largely outside of states' control. The variety of demographic and health status indicators that states use to predict spending per enrollee when setting Medicaid managed care rates illustrates the complex array of factors potentially at play. The ability to reliably calculate each state's per-enrollee Medicaid spending is a prerequisite for understanding the extent of and reasons for variation among states in such spending. Better information about Medicaid expenditures is needed in order to do so. GAO has previously recommended that CMS take steps to improve states' reporting of supplemental payments, among other steps to improve accountability and transparency for supplemental payments, and that Congress consider requiring CMS to take such steps. CMS has taken some steps to improve state reporting of these payments and is in the process of implementing a project to improve and expand MSIS. Until better information about Medicaid spending per enrollee is available, it will not be possible to quantify the effects of particular drivers of spending growth, to identify spending that is unnecessary for covering the health service needs of Medicaid enrollees, or to evaluate the effectiveness of potential approaches to curtailing Medicaid spending and how such approaches may affect program objectives.

Agency Comments

We provided the Secretary of Health and Human Services with a draft of this report. The Department of Health and Human Services provided technical comments, which we incorporated as appropriate.

Carolyn L. Yocom
Director, Health Care

APPENDIX I: DATA AND METHODOLOGY FOR ESTIMATES OF MEDICAID SPENDING PER ENROLLEE

This appendix describes the methodology we used to examine what Centers for Medicare & Medicaid Services (CMS) data show about variation among states in Medicaid spending per enrollee. We developed state-specific estimates of Medicaid spending per enrollee for fiscal year 2008 using Medicaid enrollment data and combined federal and state expenditure data provided by the CMS Office of the Actuary (OACT). Specifically, we obtained from OACT (1) enrollment data showing the number of full-year-equivalent enrollees, by state and eligibility group, which OACT calculates using data in the Medicaid Statistical Information System (MSIS); and (2) expenditure data broken out by state, eligibility group, and service category. Both enrollment and expenditure data include all enrollees, regardless of the scope of benefits offered.

OACT develops its expenditure estimates using data from two sources—the CMS-64 data system and MSIS—in order to exploit the different strengths of these two sources. CMS-64 data are regarded as the most accurate and comprehensive source of information on state Medicaid expenditures, in part because these data are reviewed by CMS and used to reimburse states for their federal shares of Medicaid expenditures. The CMS-64 data system provides expenditure data at the aggregate level, such as a state's total expenditures for such categories of services as inpatient hospital services and prescription drugs, as well as data on expenditures that are not linked to specific enrollees, such as Disproportionate Share Hospital (DSH) payments and other supplemental payments, which we refer to as non-DSH supplemental payments.[1] However, the CMS-64 data system provides no information on the amount of spending attributable to specific enrollees or eligibility groups. In contrast, MSIS provides detailed, individual-level enrollment and claims data, including data on expenditures for specific services provided to specific enrollees.[2] However, MSIS expenditure data are not considered as reliable as CMS-64 data, because they are not reviewed for use in determining the federal share of Medicaid expenditures. MSIS data are also less complete than CMS-64 data, in that they lack information on expenditures that are not linked to specific enrollees. These expenditures include drug rebates, which effectively reduce states' expenditures for drugs, as well as DSH and non-DSH supplemental payments.

OACT's expenditure estimates reflect the total spending reported in the CMS-64 data system, distributed across eligibility groups and service categories, as reported in MSIS. To develop these estimates, OACT obtains from the CMS-64 data system an annual summary report called the Base Financial Management Report, which shows expenditures for the year by category of service and also includes information on any changes states made to their quarterly expenditure reports for prior periods, such as adjustments and collections. 3 From MSIS, OACT obtains tabulations of expenditures by service category and eligibility group. To combine the data from these two sources, OACT crosswalks the service categories in the CMS-64 annual summary report to the more detailed service categories in the MSIS data, and then distributes the spending reported in the CMS-64 annual summary report across eligibility groups accordingly. For example, if disabled enrollees accounted for 50 percent of the inpatient care expenditures reported in MSIS by a given state, OACT would assign to these enrollees 50 percent of the inpatient care expenditures reported in that state's CMS-64 Base Financial Management Report. These expenditure estimates do not include states' administrative costs. DSH payments, adjustments, and collections are all reported as separate line items.

To estimate overall Medicaid spending per enrollee by state for the four major eligibility groups—children, adults, disabled, and aged—we collapsed some of the eligibility groups by which the OACT enrollment and expenditure data were broken out and then totaled the expenditures attributed to each of the four groups in each state.[4] To each group's total, we then added a share of state DSH payments. Although these payments do not represent expenditures on individual enrollees, we included them in estimates of spending per enrollee, in order to avoid skewing comparisons among states by excluding one type of supplemental payment while including another. In fiscal year 2008, states were required to separately report DSH payments in their CMS-64 quarterly reports, but lines to separately report non-DSH supplemental payments were not added to the CMS-64 until fiscal year 2010.[5] In fiscal year 2008, these payments were folded into the spending reported for related services. (For example, some non-DSH supplemental payments to hospitals could be folded into spending for inpatient or outpatient care.) Because it was therefore not possible to exclude non-DSH supplemental payments and because some states appear to use these payments more than DSH payments, while others appear to do the reverse, we included both types of supplemental payments in our estimates.

We distributed DSH payments among eligibility groups based on each group's share of state spending for relevant services. Specifically, we distributed inpatient DSH payments based on spending for services provided in these facilities (hospital inpatient and outpatient services), and mental health facility DSH payments based on spending for mental health facilities, nursing facilities, and public and private intermediate care facilities for individuals with intellectual disability. [6] For example, if children accounted for 30 percent of total spending for hospital inpatient and outpatient services in a state, we assigned 30 percent of the state's inpatient DSH payments to that eligibility group. We did not distribute adjustments or collections among eligibility groups or include them in our estimates of overall spending per enrollee because these amounts could apply to spending from prior years. Instead, we report the total adjustments and collections for each state as a separate dollar amount and as a percentage of the state's total expenditures for the year.

To assess the reliability of the data, we reviewed documentation for the OACT estimates and for MSIS and CMS-64 data, interviewed CMS officials knowledgeable about these data sources, and compared our estimates to those from other data sources. On the basis of this assessment, we excluded two states from certain analyses because of significant errors or omissions in the data they reported to CMS for fiscal year 2008. We excluded Massachusetts from all analyses of state Medicaid spending because, according to CMS officials, fiscal year 2008 enrollment data for the state mistakenly included information on many individuals who were not eligible for Medicaid and were instead covered with state funds.

We excluded Maine from analyses of state Medicaid spending at the eligibility-group level, because the state was unable to report spending by service category, which OACT uses to estimate state spending by eligibility group. We determined that for the rest of the states the data were sufficiently reliable for our purposes.

APPENDIX II: ESTIMATED MEDICAID SPENDING PER ENROLLEE BY STATE

Table 1 illustrates state variation in estimated Medicaid spending per enrollee—for enrollees overall, and for the four major Medicaid eligibility groups—children, adults, disabled, and aged.

Our analysis of expenditure data from CMS-64 annual summary reports and enrollment and expenditure data from the Medicaid Statistical Information System suggests wide variation across states in Medicaid spending per enrollee—estimated overall spending per enrollee ranged from about $3,800 in California to about $11,700 in Rhode Island in fiscal year 2008.

Table 1. Estimated Medicaid Spending per Enrollee for All Enrollees and for Each Eligibility Group, by State, Fiscal Year 2008

	Estimated Medicaid spending per enrollee				
State	All enrollees	Children	Adults	Disabled	Aged
Alabama	$5,410	$2,890	$3,556	$8,870	$9,882
Alaska	11,111	4,298	7,920	31,835	25,780
Arizona	6,331	3,344	6,086	17,080	11,064
Arkansas	5,913	2,606	2,031	12,721	15,205
California	3,838	1,702	1,480	13,089	9,938
Colorado	7,827	2,802	6,132	20,776	18,022
Connecticut	9,659	3,226	3,765	30,396	26,067
Delaware	7,333	2,937	5,989	18,902	17,364
District of Columbia	10,510	4,119	6,006	23,220	27,322
Florida	6,577	2,288	5,314	14,510	11,345
Georgia	6,062	2,562	8,115	11,844	12,117
Hawaii	6,756	2,306	4,971	20,802	14,000
Idaho	7,561	2,474	8,540	19,337	14,029
Illinois	5,799	2,227	3,935	18,910	11,261
Indiana	8,052	2,521	4,995	23,213	21,757
Iowa	7,608	2,535	3,490	20,017	19,828
Kansas	8,702	2,644	5,966	20,217	18,870
Kentucky	7,003	2,924	6,736	11,082	13,450
Louisiana	6,593	2,123	5,471	16,911	11,533
Maine[a]	7,452	—	—	—	—
Maryland	9,548	3,630	5,871	22,795	20,950
Massachusetts[b]	—	—	—	—	—
Michigan	6,209	2,075	5,672	14,388	19,632
Minnesota	11,308	4,157	5,229	31,570	24,505
Mississippi	5,827	2,444	3,983	10,441	12,140
Missouri	8,695	3,815	5,227	20,959	17,162
Montana	9,613	3,112	7,031	20,682	28,564
Nebraska	8,742	3,394	4,717	21,654	21,179
Nevada	7,026	3,006	5,029	17,876	12,729
New Hampshire	10,854	3,905	8,508	25,237	29,613
New Jersey	11,612	2,758	7,908	28,393	22,817

	Estimated Medicaid spending per enrollee				
State	All enrollees	Children	Adults	Disabled	Aged
New Mexico	7,133	3,603	5,251	22,658	12,314
New York	11,310	2,873	5,635	32,185	29,734
North Carolina	7,462	2,755	5,938	17,401	13,449
North Dakota	10,535	2,902	5,087	25,087	25,213
Ohio	7,510	2,105	4,432	17,421	21,800
Oklahoma	6,376	2,614	5,119	16,081	13,375
Oregon	8,191	2,704	6,760	16,947	19,463
Pennsylvania	9,030	3,026	5,019	14,175	27,207
Rhode Island	11,680	5,107	5,982	22,972	21,574
South Carolina	6,401	2,818	4,941	13,247	13,704
South Dakota	7,064	2,146	6,031	19,587	15,559
Tennessee	5,827	2,644	5,338	10,262	12,694
Texas	6,540	3,345	7,131	15,680	10,495
Utah	7,882	3,723	4,857	23,896	14,468
Vermont	7,706	5,877	5,708	13,984	10,981
Virginia	7,554	2,622	5,494	17,251	14,693
Washington	6,785	2,376	5,107	17,432	19,207
West Virginia	7,037	2,467	5,759	11,584	15,863
Wisconsin	6,432	1,902	3,329	17,389	11,262
Wyoming	8,358	3,250	6,756	24,644	21,662
State average	$7,847	$2,973	$5,497	$19,135	$17,609

Source: GAO analysis of Centers for Medicare & Medicaid Services data. | GAO-14-456

Notes: Estimates of spending per enrollee include federal and state spending on regular Medicaid payments to providers and managed care plans for covered services provided to enrollees as well as Disproportionate Share Hospital (DSH) and non-DSH supplemental payments, but do not include administrative costs. Estimates also do not reflect states' subsequent changes, including adjustments or collections, to the spending originally reported for this year. Enrollment is measured in terms of fullyear-equivalent enrollees. Both enrollment and expenditure data include all enrollees, regardless of the scope of benefits offered. State average spending per enrollee represents the sum of each state's estimated spending per enrollee divided by the number of states. For purposes of this table we refer to the District of Columbia as a state.

[a]We excluded Maine from eligibility-group level estimates because the state was unable to report spending by service category for fiscal year 2008.

[b]We excluded Massachusetts from the estimates because of errors in fiscal year 2008 CMS data for this state.

APPENDIX III: TOTAL MEDICAID SPENDING AND ADJUSTMENTS AND COLLECTIONS BY STATE

States are required to report to CMS each quarter any collections or adjustments to the Medicaid spending they previously reported. In one of the annual summary reports available from the CMS-64 data system, the adjustments and collections reported by a state that year are summed by type—for example, adjustments increasing claims—and reported as line items separate from other reported spending amounts.[1] The reported sums may include adjustments and collections applicable to spending for the current year as well as prior years.[2] For six states, the adjustments and collections reported in fiscal year 2008—an unknown amount of which was applicable to that year's spending—represented 5 percent or more of the total spending reported for that year. Table 2 shows the total spending states reported for fiscal year 2008, as well as the total adjustments and collections they reported that year, and the percentage of total spending that adjustments and collections represented.

Table 2. Total Medicaid Spending and Adjustments and Collections Reported in Fiscal Year 2008

State	Total spending	Adjustments and collections	Adjustments andcollections as apercentage oftotal spending
Alabama	$4,065,658,513	($3,403,747)	-0.1
Alaska	962,595,105	(72,726,013)	-7.6
Arizona	7,285,798,764	217,986,033	3.0
Arkansas	3,320,009,018	(95,445,204)	-2.9
California	31,039,145,327	7,546,974,470	24.3
Colorado	3,186,825,239	(34,849,295)	-1.1
Connecticut	4,515,843,293	(98,177,252)	-2.2
Delaware	1,103,519,563	(1,363,880)	-0.1
District of Columbia	1,459,889,715	(31,962,688)	-2.2
Florida	14,674,721,802	(73,161,543)	-0.5
Georgia	7,654,184,658	(390,248,341)	-5.1
Hawaii	1,222,550,545	(20,392,992)	-1.7
Idaho	1,220,236,237	(32,553,305)	-2.7
Illinois	11,730,832,868	(263,433,221)	-2.2
Indiana	6,679,844,413	(565,918,130)	-8.5
Iowa	2,834,135,869	(56,770,325)	-2.0

State	Total spending	Adjustments and collections	Adjustments andcollections as apercentage oftotal spending
Kansas	2,338,692,399	(114,140,708)	-4.9
Kentucky	4,781,853,623	(90,229,659)	-1.9
Louisiana	6,065,775,886	(234,590,878)	-3.9
Maine	2,186,642,908	47,453,663	2.2
Maryland	5,789,864,630	(151,620,736)	-2.6
Massachusetts[a]	—	—	—
Michigan	9,763,205,475	31,721,058	0.3
Minnesota	6,963,611,523	(79,838,444)	-1.1
Mississippi	3,534,943,883	258,504,898	7.3
Missouri	7,065,432,032	(78,221,022)	-1.1
Montana	780,125,095	(10,369,615)	-1.3
Nebraska	1,585,314,119	(32,318,151)	-2.0
Nevada	1,308,662,237	3,712,625	0.3
New Hampshire	1,256,516,384	(16,206,643)	-1.3
New Jersey	9,390,013,827	(36,195,450)	-0.4
New Mexico	3,051,859,421	(27,864,999)	-0.9
New York	46,004,929,844	258,553,798	0.6
North Carolina	9,984,558,550	(370,706,876)	-3.7
North Dakota	555,283,315	(26,625,586)	-4.8
Ohio	12,208,921,164	(16,039,100)	-0.1
Oklahoma	3,525,551,862	(105,739,641)	-3.0
Oregon	3,188,916,042	(11,560,143)	-0.4
Pennsylvania	16,137,965,265	48,605,230	0.3
Rhode Island	1,846,481,589	(43,086,140)	-2.3
South Carolina	4,435,472,577	(209,104,361)	-4.7
South Dakota	672,641,093	(20,933,097)	-3.1
Tennessee	7,296,597,016	(162,724,231)	-2.2
Texas	20,942,941,607	154,234,451	0.7
Utah	1,570,682,903	(81,216,971)	-5.2
Vermont	1,034,050,857	45,268,884	4.4
Virginia	5,361,612,424	(33,874,206)	-0.6
Washington	6,381,271,503	(139,384,829)	-2.2
West Virginia	2,279,677,025	(16,083,970)	-0.7
Wisconsin	5,103,833,259	(182,497,433)	-3.6
Wyoming	485,726,260	(1,714,150)	-0.4
State Average	**$6,356,868,371**	**$91,594,443**	**-1.1%**

Source: GAO analysis of Centers for Medicare & Medicaid Services data. | GAO-14-456

Notes: Total spending includes federal and state spending on regular Medicaid payments to providers and managed care plans for covered services provided to enrollees as well as Disproportionate Share Hospital (DSH) and non-DSH supplemental payments and does not include adjustments, collections, or administrative costs. For purposes of this table we refer to the District of Columbia as a state.

[a]We excluded Massachusetts from the estimates because of errors in fiscal year 2008 CMS data for this state.

Appendix IV: Estimated Medicaid Spending per Enrollee, by State, Using Two Possible Methods to Distribute DSH Payments

Federal Medicaid law requires states to make DSH payments to qualifying hospitals that serve large numbers of Medicaid and uninsured low-income patients. States are required to report to CMS separate data on the two types of DSH payments: payments to inpatient hospitals and payments to inpatient mental health facilities.[1] We included DSH payments in our estimates of spending per enrollee, and compared two possible methods of distributing these payments among eligibility groups. For the first method—the one used in our estimates of spending per enrollee—we distributed DSH payments among eligibility groups based on each group's share of state spending for services delivered in the types of facilities that are potentially eligible for DSH payments. Specifically, we distributed inpatient DSH payments based on spending for services provided in these facilities (hospital inpatient and outpatient services), and mental health facility DSH payments based on spending for mental health facilities, nursing facilities, and public and private intermediate care facilities for individuals with intellectual disability. For the second method, we distributed DSH payments among eligibility groups based on each group's share of total spending. We found that for some eligibility groups in some states, the method used to distribute DSH payments significantly affected estimates of spending per enrollee. Table 3 shows estimated Medicaid spending per enrollee by state and by eligibility group, for fiscal year 2008, using these two different methods to distribute DSH payments.

Table 3. Estimated Medicaid Spending per Enrollee Using Two Possible Methods to Distribute Disproportionate Share Hospital (DSH) Payments, by Eligibility Group and State, Fiscal Year 2008

	With DSH payments distributed across groups based on share of spending for relevant services[a]				With DSH payments distributed across groups based on share of total spending[b]			
State	Children	Adults	Disabled	Aged	Children	Adults	Disabled	Aged
Alabama	$2,890	$3,556	$8,870	$9,882	$2,995	$2,533	$8,972	$10,450
Alaska	4,298	7,920	31,835	25,780	4,318	7,983	31,844	25,447
Arizona	3,344	6,086	17,080	11,064	3,351	6,091	17,103	10,936
Arkansas	2,606	2,031	12,721	15,205	2,603	2,024	12,722	15,227
California	1,702	1,480	13,089	9,938	1,711	1,383	13,088	10,329
Colorado	2,802	6,132	20,776	18,022	2,737	5,660	20,970	18,772
Connecticut	3,226	3,765	30,396	26,067	3,263	3,797	30,194	26,064
Delaware	2,937	5,989	18,902	17,364	2,951	6,018	18,914	17,134
District of Columbia	4,119	6,006	23,220	27,322	4,202	6,132	22,721	28,169
Florida	2,288	5,314	14,510	11,345	2,287	5,273	14,550	11,329
Georgia	2,562	8,115	11,844	12,117	2,589	8,062	11,548	12,660
Hawaii	2,306	4,971	20,802	14,000	2,334	4,943	20,300	14,558
Idaho	2,474	8,540	19,337	14,029	2,451	8,327	19,418	14,231
Illinois	2,227	3,935	18,910	11,261	2,230	3,940	18,906	11,236
Indiana	2,521	4,995	23,213	21,757	2,574	5,127	22,775	22,016
Iowa	2,535	3,490	20,017	19,828	2,525	3,462	20,037	19,913
Kansas	2,644	5,966	20,217	18,870	2,677	6,023	20,259	18,558
Kentucky	2,924	6,736	11,082	13,450	2,945	6,593	11,073	13,572
Louisiana	2,123	5,471	16,911	11,533	2,037	4,825	16,920	12,868
Maine[c]	—	—	—	—	—	—	—	—
Maryland	3,630	5,871	22,795	20,950	3,643	5,907	22,841	20,665
Massachusetts[d]	—	—	—	—	—	—	—	—
Michigan	2,075	5,672	14,388	19,632	2,073	5,687	14,465	19,418
Minnesota	4,157	5,229	31,570	24,505	4,155	5,190	31,400	24,864
Mississippi	2,444	3,983	10,441	12,140	2,396	3,794	10,416	12,664
Missouri	3,815	5,227	20,959	17,162	3,892	5,335	20,821	16,824
Montana	3,112	7,031	20,682	28,564	3,076	6,894	20,663	29,065
Nebraska	3,394	4,717	21,654	21,179	3,374	4,630	21,658	21,398
Nevada	3,006	5,029	17,876	12,729	3,041	4,884	17,506	13,376
New Hampshire	3,905	8,508	25,237	29,613	3,618	6,385	26,310	31,736
New Jersey	2,758	7,908	28,393	22,817	2,835	8,005	28,203	22,740
New Mexico	3,603	5,251	22,658	12,314	3,597	5,228	22,693	12,372
New York	2,873	5,635	32,185	29,734	2,809	5,447	32,225	30,606

Table 3. (Continued)

State	With DSH payments distributed across groups based on share of spending for relevant services[a]				With DSH payments distributed across groups based on share of total spending[b]			
	Children	Adults	Disabled	Aged	Children	Adults	Disabled	Aged
North Carolina	2,755	5,938	17,401	13,449	2,770	5,824	17,453	13,442
North Dakota	2,902	5,087	25,087	25,213	2,904	5,091	25,099	25,186
Ohio	2,105	4,432	17,421	21,800	2,105	4,432	17,421	21,800
Oklahoma	2,614	5,119	16,081	13,375	2,602	5,060	16,103	13,489
Oregon	2,704	6,760	16,947	19,463	2,699	6,734	16,991	19,456
Pennsylvania	3,026	5,019	14,175	27,207	3,053	4,929	14,266	27,010
Rhode Island	5,107	5,982	22,972	21,574	5,263	6,217	22,111	22,530
South Carolina	2,818	4,941	13,247	13,704	2,813	4,702	13,223	14,304
South Dakota	2,146	6,031	19,587	15,559	2,147	6,032	19,599	15,531
Tennessee	2,644	5,338	10,262	12,694	2,644	5,326	10,253	12,766
Texas	3,345	7,131	15,680	10,495	3,369	6,936	15,531	10,723
Utah	3,723	4,857	23,896	14,468	3,706	4,806	23,989	14,578
Vermont	5,877	5,708	13,984	10,981	5,955	5,532	13,924	11,272
Virginia	2,622	5,494	17,251	14,693	2,617	5,411	17,194	14,908
Washington	2,376	5,107	17,432	19,207	2,463	5,214	17,112	19,027
West Virginia	2,467	5,759	11,584	15,863	2,507	5,762	11,505	15,919
Wisconsin	1,902	3,329	17,389	11,262	1,895	3,325	17,297	11,398
Wyoming	3,250	6,756	24,644	21,662	3,249	6,755	24,645	21,665
State average	$2,973	$5,497	$19,135	$17,609	$2,981	$5,381	$19,086	$17,841

Source: GAO analysis of Centers for Medicare & Medicaid Services data. | GAO-14-456

Notes: Estimates of spending per enrollee include federal and state spending on regular Medicaid payments to providers and managed care plans for covered services provided to enrollees, as well DSH and non-DSH supplemental payments, but do not include administrative costs. Estimates also do not reflect states' subsequent changes, including adjustments or collections, to the spending originally reported for this year. Enrollment is measured in terms of full-year-equivalent enrollees. Both enrollment and expenditure data include all enrollees, regardless of the scope of benefits offered. State average spending per enrollee represents the sum of each state's estimated spending per enrollee divided by the number of states. For purposes of this table we refer to the District of Columbia as a state.

[a]For this method, we distributed DSH payments among eligibility groups based on each group's share of state spending for relevant services. Specifically, we distributed inpatient DSH payments based on spending for hospital inpatient and outpatient services and mental health facility DSH payments based on spending for mental health facilities, nursing facilities, and public and private intermediate care facilities for individuals with intellectual disability.

[b]For this method, we distributed DSH payments among eligibility groups based on each group's share of total spending.

[c]We excluded Maine from eligibility-group level estimates because the state was unable to report spending by service category for fiscal year 2008.

[d]We excluded Massachusetts from the estimates because of errors in fiscal year 2008 CMS data for this state.

APPENDIX V: STATE DSH PAYMENTS AS A PERCENTAGE OF TOTAL STATE MEDICAID SPENDING AND EFFECT ON OVERALL SPENDING PER ENROLLEE

Federal Medicaid law requires states to make DSH payments to qualifying hospitals that serve large numbers of Medicaid and uninsured low-income patients. DSH payments represent varying proportions of states' total Medicaid spending, ranging from 0 to 18 percent. Thus the effect of including these payments in estimates of state spending per enrollee also varies. Table 4 presents DSH payments as a percentage of each state's total Medicaid spending for fiscal year 2008, as well as overall state spending per enrollee excluding and including DSH payments.

Table 4. Disproportionate Share Hospital (DSH) Payments as a Percentage of Total State Medicaid Spending and Overall Spending per Enrollee Excluding and Including DSH Payments, Fiscal Year 2008

State	DSH payments as percentage of total state Medicaid spending	Overall spending per enrollee	
		Excluding DSH payments	Including DSH payments
Alabama	10.5%	$4,840	$5,410
Alaska	1.6	10,931	11,111
Arizona	1.6	6,231	6,331
Arkansas	0.3	5,898	5,913
California	6.1	3,604	3,838
Colorado	5.2	7,420	7,827
Connecticut	5.9	9,091	9,659
Delaware	0.5	7,296	7,333
District of Columbia	4.8	10,009	10,510
Florida	2.3	6,429	6,577
Georgia	5.2	5,744	6,062
Hawaii	2.5	6,585	6,756

Table 4. (Continued)

State	DSH payments as percentage of total state Medicaid spending	Overall spending per enrollee	
		Excluding DSH payments	Including DSH payments
Idaho	1.8	7,424	7,561
Illinois	1.7	5,703	5,799
Indiana	7.0	7,492	8,052
Iowa	0.6	7,566	7,608
Kansas	3.5	8,402	8,702
Kentucky	4.1	6,716	7,003
Louisiana	16.6	5,498	6,593
Maine	2.3	7,281	7,452
Maryland	1.9	9,365	9,548
Massachusetts[a]	—	—	—
Michigan	4.5	5,927	6,209
Minnesota	1.7	11,120	11,308
Mississippi	5.1	5,532	5,827
Missouri	9.9	7,831	8,695
Montana	2.0	9,422	9,613
Nebraska	1.7	8,595	8,742
Nevada	6.3	6,582	7,026
New Hampshire	17.8	8,926	10,854
New Jersey	16.3	9,721	11,612
New Mexico	0.9	7,072	7,133
New York	4.8	10,764	11,310
North Carolina	4.3	7,144	7,462
North Dakota	0.2	10,511	10,535
Ohio	0.0	7,510	7,510
Oklahoma	1.4	6,285	6,376
Oregon	1.9	8,036	8,191
Pennsylvania	4.6	8,613	9,030
Rhode Island	6.4	10,938	11,680
South Carolina	10.0	5,763	6,401
South Dakota	0.2	7,050	7,064
Tennessee	0.6	5,792	5,827
Texas	6.5	6,117	6,540
Utah	1.3	7,780	7,882
Vermont	3.5	7,439	7,706
Virginia	3.4	7,294	7,554
Washington	5.1	6,437	6,785
West Virginia	3.2	6,812	7,037

State	DSH payments as percentage of total state Medicaid spending	Overall spending per enrollee Excluding DSH payments	Including DSH payments
Wisconsin	1.7	6,320	6,432
Wyoming	0.0	8,356	8,358
State average	4.2%	$7,504	$7,847

Source: GAO analysis of Centers for Medicare & Medicaid Services data. | GAO-14-456

Notes: Total state spending and spending per enrollee include federal and state spending on regular Medicaid payments to providers and managed care plans for covered services provided to enrollees as well as DSH and non-DSH supplemental payments. Estimates do not reflect states' subsequent changes, including adjustments or collections, to the spending originally reported for this year and do not include administrative costs. Enrollment is measured in terms of full-year-equivalent enrollees. Both enrollment and expenditure data include all enrollees, regardless of the scope of benefits offered. The state averages represent the sum of state percentages or state spending per enrollee divided by the number of states. For the purposes of this table, we refer to the District of Columbia as a state.

[a]We excluded Massachusetts because of errors in fiscal year 2008 CMS data for this state.

APPENDIX VI: DISTRIBUTION OF STATE MEDICAID ENROLLEES BY ELIGIBILITY GROUP

Table 5 illustrates that the distribution of Medicaid enrollees in each of the four major Medicaid eligibility groups (children, adults, disabled, and aged)—a program characteristic known to influence overall per-enrollee Medicaid spending—varied widely by state in calendar year 2008.

Table 5. Distribution of Medicaid Enrollees by Eligibility Group and State, Calendar Year 2008

State	Percentage of Medicaid Enrollees[a] Children	Adults	Disabled	Aged
Alabama	49.5%	15.0%	24.3%	11.1%
Alaska	60.0	21.3	12.9	5.7
Arizona	45.2	40.0	9.2	5.5
Arkansas	57.3	16.1	17.5	9.1
California	40.0	41.8	10.8	7.4
Colorado	58.4	16.8	15.3	9.4

Table 5. (Continued)

State	Percentage of Medicaid Enrollees[a]			
	Children	Adults	Disabled	Aged
Connecticut	51.9	23.9	12.3	11.9
Delaware	42.7	38.5	11.8	7.0
District of Columbia	47.3	23.3	22.7	6.7
Florida	50.3	19.3	18.1	12.3
Georgia	57.4	16.6	17.9	8.1
Hawaii	46.3	33.6	10.7	9.4
Idaho	63.4	12.6	16.7	7.3
Illinois	55.9	25.1	13.4	5.6
Indiana	58.0	20.6	14.0	7.5
Iowa	48.4	28.1	15.0	8.5
Kansas	55.8	14.6	19.6	10.0
Kentucky	49.1	15.3	25.1	10.6
Louisiana	58.2	15.8	16.9	9.1
Maine	37.1	29.5	17.2	16.2
Maryland	56.2	21.0	16.2	6.6
Massachusetts	33.0	40.3	16.2	10.5
Michigan	53.8	23.8	15.6	6.7
Minnesota	48.4	25.5	14.7	11.5
Mississippi	49.6	16.7	23.4	10.3
Missouri	55.7	17.2	18.2	8.9
Montana	54.4	18.5	18.4	8.7
Nebraska	61.2	16.1	13.7	8.9
Nevada	56.1	19.9	15.0	8.9
New Hampshire	59.7	13.6	16.7	10.0
New Jersey	51.4	20.5	16.9	11.1
New Mexico	57.5	25.5	12.3	4.7
New York	38.9	36.8	15.0	9.3
North Carolina	53.2	19.3	17.2	10.2
North Dakota	51.4	21.2	15.0	12.4
Ohio	53.1	21.5	17.3	8.1
Oklahoma	60.7	16.7	14.5	8.1
Oregon	50.1	23.5	16.5	9.9
Pennsylvania	45.1	19.8	24.5	10.6
Rhode Island	45.1	24.6	20.9	9.5
South Carolina	52.2	21.9	17.4	8.5
South Dakota	62.2	15.4	14.5	7.9
Tennessee	49.7	20.2	23.2	6.9
Texas	62.2	14.1	13.6	10.1
Utah	55.2	26.8	13.2	4.8

State	Percentage of Medicaid Enrollees[a]			
	Children	Adults	Disabled	Aged
Vermont	38.2	37.1	14.0	10.7
Virginia	56.1	15.4	18.0	10.5
Washington	54.9	21.9	15.7	7.6
West Virginia	47.4	14.6	28.7	9.3
Wisconsin	43.9	29.4	14.5	12.2
Wyoming	65.3	14.3	13.3	7.1
State average	52.0%	22.4%	16.6%	9.0%

Source: GAO analysis of Centers for Medicare & Medicaid Services (CMS) data. | GAO-14-456

Notes: State average represents the sum of the state percentages divided by the number of states. For purposes of this table, we refer to the District of Columbia as a state.

[a]Based on CMS *Medicaid Analytic eXtract 2008 Chartbook* data for calendar year 2008.

APPENDIX VII: SELECTED FACTORS THAT ARE KNOWN TO INFLUENCE HEALTH CARE SPENDING, BY STATE

Tables 6 and 7 illustrate state variation on selected factors that are known to influence health care spending, such as indicators of enrollee health services needs and scope of benefits received.

Table 6. State Variation on Selected Factors That Can Influence Health Care Spending for Aged Medicaid Enrollees, Fiscal or Calendar Year 2008

State	Percentage of aged Medicaid enrollees who were 85 and older[a]	Percentage of aged Medicaid enrollees receiving long-term care services[a]	Percentage of aged Medicaid enrollees ever institutionalized during the year[b,c]
Alabama	23.7	23.5	17.8
Alaska	16.8	39.7	8.2
Arizonad	17.9	—	—
Arkansas	23.1	34.6	21.9
California	18.3	30.3	10.2
Colorado	22.2	45.0	21.9
Connecticut	30.7	51.1	35.7
Delaware	23.7	26.6	21.8

Table 6. (Continued)

State	Percentage of aged Medicaid enrollees who were 85 and older[a]	Percentage of aged Medicaid enrollees receiving long-term care services[a]	Percentage of aged Medicaid enrollees ever institutionalized during the year[b,c]
District of Columbia	21.2	27.7	20.4
Florida	21.1	18.4	14.2
Georgia	22.4	23.4	20.4
Hawaii	22.2	23.3	15.9
Idaho	22.6	47.4	22.2
Illinois	27.0	33.4	28.2
Indiana	24.4	37.9	36.3
Iowa	30.2	65.6	37.2
Kansas	28.8	54.2	35.0
Kentucky	22.7	32.1	21.4
Louisiana	19.1	25.2	20.3
Mainee	21.9	—	—
Maryland	24.8	32.0	28.9
Massachusettsf	—	—	23.6
Michigan	22.7	40.9	26.3
Minnesota	33.4	36.0	23.9
Mississippi	23.3	27.3	21.1
Missouri	24.5	48.4	30.8
Montana	31.3	52.9	42.5
Nebraska	29.7	48.4	37.3
Nevada	16.6	28.2	13.7
New Hampshire	30.9	51.0	41.0
New Jersey	29.9	38.3	26.0
New Mexicod	22.4	—	—
New York	26.3	38.0	22.0
North Carolina	22.7	40.5	18.9
North Dakota	36.8	54.9	46.1
Ohio	23.7	47.4	34.9
Oklahoma	20.1	44.4	25.5
Oregon	21.3	44.9	13.9
Pennsylvania	24.5	32.5	29.6
Rhode Island	33.0	38.2	35.8
South Carolina	23.6	29.1	18.7
South Dakota	38.9	49.6	42.5
Tennessee	24.8	24.7	23.4
Texas	19.1	35.9	17.0

State	Percentage of aged Medicaid enrollees who were 85 and older[a]	Percentage of aged Medicaid enrollees receiving long-term care services[a]	Percentage of aged Medicaid enrollees ever institutionalized during the year[b,c]
Utah	19.4	28.7	23.3
Vermont	26.3	27.3	16.4
Virginia	21.9	31.4	21.2
Washington	20.8	45.8	16.1
West Virginia	18.1	29.3	24.3
Wisconsind	33.2	—	—
Wyoming	26.4	48.7	35.7
State average	24.6	37.7	24.5

Source: GAO analysis of Centers for Medicare & Medicaid Services (CMS) data. | GAO-14-456

Notes: State average represents the sum of state percentages, divided by the number of states. For purposes of this table, we refer to the District of Columbia as a state.

[a]Based on CMS Medicaid Statistical Information System (MSIS) data for fiscal year 2008. [b]Based on CMS *Medicaid Analytic eXtract 2008 Chartbook* data for calendar year 2008.

[c]Institutionalized enrollees include those receiving Medicaid-covered services in nursing homes, intermediate care facilities for individuals with intellectual disability, mental hospitals for the aged, or inpatient psychiatric facilities for those under age 21 at any time in 2008.

[d]Excluded from long-term care service use and ever-institutionalized data because more than 2 percent of all enrollees in the state—and therefore likely a higher percentage of aged enrollees— received long-term care services through managed care plans and therefore were not represented in the fee-for-service data used to identify enrollees who received long-term care services during the year.

[e]Excluded from long-term care service use and ever-institutionalized data because of the state's inability to accurately report data related to service use in 2008.

[f] Excluded from percentage of aged who were 85 years or older and long-term care service use data because of errors in fiscal year 2008 CMS MSIS data.

Table 7. State Variation on Selected Factors That Can Influence Health Care Spending for Children and Adults, Fiscal or Calendar Year 2008

State	Percentage of child Medicaid enrollees in foster care[a]	Percentage of adult Medicaid enrollees receiving only family planning benefits [b]	Percentage of adult state residents who reported being obese[c]	Percentage of adult state residents who reported smoking tobacco [c]
Alabama	2%	53%	32%	22%
Alaska	5	0	27	21
Arizona	2	1	26	17
Arkansas	2	61	30	22
California	4	55	24	14
Colorado	6	0	19	18
Connecticut	2	0	21	16
Delaware	3	4	28	18
District of Columbia	6	0	22	16
Florida	3	7	25	18
Georgia	4	0	28	19
Hawaii	7	0	23	16
Idaho	3	0	25	17
Illinois	5	5	27	20
Indiana	3	0	27	24
Iowa	5	20	27	19
Kansas	8	0	28	18
Kentucky	4	0	30	26
Louisiana	2	24	29	22
Maine	4	0	26	19
Maryland	5	15	27	16
Massachusettsd	—	0	22	16
Michigan	4	10	30	20
Minnesota	3	15	25	17
Mississippi	1	30	33	23
Missouri	6	7	29	24
Montana	7	0	24	18
Nebraska	11	0	27	18
Nevada	7	0	26	22
New Hampshire	3	0	25	17
New Jersey	6	0	24	16
New Mexico	2	17	26	19
New York	3	3	25	18
North Carolina	3	12	30	21

State	Percentage of child Medicaid enrollees in foster carea	Percentage of adult Medicaid enrollees receiving only family planning benefits b	Percentage of adult state residents who reported being obesec	Percentage of adult state residents who reported smoking tobacco c
North Dakota	5	0	28	19
Ohio	6	0	29	21
Oklahoma	3	19	31	25
Oregon	7	0	25	17
Pennsylvania	6	11	28	21
Rhode Island	7	1	22	17
South Carolina	3	27	31	21
South Dakota	8	0	28	18
Tennessee	3	0	31	23
Texas	2	0	29	19
Utah	6	0	23	10
Vermont	4	0	23	17
Virginia	3	6	26	18
Washington	3	31	26	16
West Virginia	4	0	32	26
Wisconsin	5	22	26	19
Wyoming	7	0	25	21
State average	4%	9%	27%	19%

Source: GAO analysis of Centers for Medicare & Medicaid Services (CMS) and Centers for Disease Control and Prevention (CDC) data. | GAO-14-456

Notes: State average represents the sum of state percentages, divided by the number of states. For purposes of this table, we refer to the District of Columbia as a state.

[a]Based on CMS Medicaid Statistical Information System (MSIS) fiscal year 2008 data.

[b]Based on CMS *Medicaid Analytic eXtract 2008 Chartbook* data for calendar year 2008. [c]Based on CDC's Behavioral Risk Factor Surveillance Survey data for calendar year 2008. [d]Excluded from foster care data because of errors in fiscal year 2008 CMS MSIS data.

End Notes

[1] States administer their individual Medicaid programs subject to approval and oversight by the Centers for Medicare & Medicaid Services (CMS), a federal agency within the Department of Health and Human Services (HHS). Medicaid serves certain categories of low-income individuals, such as children, pregnant women, parents, persons with disabilities, and persons aged 65 and older.

[2] See Congressional Budget Office, *Updated Budget Projections: 2014 to 2024* (Washington, D.C.: April 2014). Under PPACA, states are permitted to expand eligibility for Medicaid to

nonpregnant, nonelderly adults whose income does not exceed 133 percent of the federal poverty level and will receive enhanced federal funding for this newly eligible population. As of April 1, 2014, 26 states and the District of Columbia had decided to implement this expansion.

[3] See National Conference of State Legislators, *Payment Reform* (Denver, Colo.: 2013).

[4] For example, a fiscal year 2012 appropriations bill passed by the House would have made Medicaid a block grant program, and other recently proposed legislation would place per capita caps on federal Medicaid funding. Under block grant proposals, the federal government generally provides states fixed grant amounts indexed to grow at a specified rate over time. In general, such block grants would not otherwise increase to reflect changes in states' Medicaid costs and enrollment. Under per capita cap proposals, the federal government generally provides states with a specified amount of funding per enrollee, but enrollment and overall spending are not necessarily limited.

[5] For example, we previously reported that the formula used under the current financing structure is an incomplete measure to equitably allocate federal funding among states and that available data sources could be used to more equitably allocate funding. See GAO, *Medicaid: Alternative Measures Could Be Used to Allocate Funding More Equitably*, GAO-13-434 (Washington, D.C.: May 10, 2013).

[6] In this report, we use "fiscal year" to refer to the federal fiscal year, and references to Medicaid spending refer to combined federal and state expenditures.

[7] Both enrollment and expenditure data include all enrollees, regardless of the scope of benefits offered.

[8] Federal Medicaid law requires states to make DSH payments to qualifying hospitals that serve large numbers of Medicaid and uninsured low-income patients. Data in CMS's *2010 Actuarial Report on the Financial Outlook for Medicaid* indicate that, nationally, administrative costs represented about 5 percent of Medicaid outlays in fiscal year 2009.

[9] We excluded Massachusetts from all analyses of state Medicaid spending because, according to CMS officials, the state's fiscal year 2008 enrollment data included information on many individuals who were not eligible for Medicaid and were instead covered with state funds. We excluded Maine from analyses of state Medicaid spending at the eligibility-group level (children, adults, disabled, and aged), because the state was unable to accurately report spending by service category, which OACT uses to estimate state spending by eligibility group. See appendix I for more information on OACT's methodology.

[10] See CMS, *Medicaid Analytic eXtract 2008 Chartbook*, research conducted by Mathematica Policy Research (Washington, D.C.: 2012). MSIS data are available in several formats. MAX files are considered to have the highest-quality MSIS data, but also have delayed availability.

[11] The MSIS Annual Person Summary files include enrollment data and annual expenditure data for each person by type of service. The MSIS State Summary DataMart files include aggregated summary information on Medicaid enrollees, such as the number of enrollees in particular age or eligibility groups.

[12] In Arizona, New Mexico, and Wisconsin, more than 2 percent of all enrollees—and therefore likely a higher percentage of aged enrollees—received long-term care services through managed care plans and therefore were not represented in the fee-for-service data used to identify enrollees who had received long-term care services during the year. Maine was unable to accurately report spending by service category, such as long-term care services.

[13] According to CMS officials, fiscal year 2008 MSIS data for Massachusetts mistakenly included information on many individuals who were not eligible for Medicaid and were instead covered with state funds; however, the problem was corrected in MAX.

[14] We interviewed representatives from the following consulting firms: Deloitte Consulting LLP, Mercer Government Human Services Consulting, Milliman, Optumas, and PricewaterhouseCoopers LLP. We included the District of Columbia as a state.

[15] We selected three states—Arizona, Florida, and New York—that have a high proportion of their Medicaid population, including individuals in the aged or disabled eligibility groups, enrolled in managed care plans.

[16] One study estimated that, nationally, optional populations accounted for about 30 percent of Medicaid enrollment in 2007, while optional services—primarily long-term care services—accounted for about 33 percent of Medicaid expenditures. See Kaiser Commission on Medicaid and the Uninsured, *January 2012 Update: Medicaid Enrollment and Expenditures by Federal Core Requirements and State Options* (Washington, D.C.: Kaiser Family Foundation, 2012).

[17] Under Section 1115 of the Social Security Act, states may apply for and receive CMS approval for demonstration waivers that allow states to deviate from their traditional Medicaid program. Specifically, states may receive a waiver for certain Medicaid requirements and approval to claim federal matching funds for items not otherwise covered by Medicaid. For example, states may apply for a Section 1115 demonstration waiver in order to provide only family planning benefits for individuals—typically women of childbearing age—who are not otherwise eligible for Medicaid. In addition, most Medicaid enrollees who are aged 65 and older or disabled are also eligible for Medicare, the federal health insurance program that covers seniors aged 65 and older, disabled persons, and individuals with end-stage renal disease. While many of these enrollees, referred to as "dual-eligibles," qualify for the full range of Medicaid benefits provided in their state, others qualify only to receive assistance for Medicare premiums and cost-sharing.

[18] The FMAP is calculated using a statutory formula based on the state's per capita income (PCI) in relation to the national PCI: FMAP = 1.00 – 0.45 (State PCI / U.S. PCI) and may range from 50 to 83 percent. The federal government pays a larger portion of Medicaid expenditures in states with low PCI relative to the national average, and a smaller portion for states with higher PCIs.

[19] Under federal law, states may only claim federal matching funds for DSH payments made to qualifying hospitals up to the states' DSH allotments, which are based on a statutory formula and vary across the states. Individual hospitals may only receive DSH payments up to their hospital-specific limit. States also make DSH payments out of their allotment to institutions for mental disease and other mental health facilities that provide inpatient services. However, federal law limits the total amount of federal matching funds that states may claim for DSH payments made to these mental health facilities. 42 U.S.C. § 1396r-4.

[20] Unlike DSH payments, non-DSH supplemental payments are not required to be made under federal law or regulations. One type of non-DSH supplemental payment, also known as upper payment limit payments, can be made to providers above the standard Medicaid payment rates but within the upper payment limit, which is the estimated amount that Medicare pays for comparable services. In addition, under upper payment limit arrangements, payments are subject to aggregate limits by provider type, but there are not firm dollar limits on individual providers or at the state level. See 42 C.F.R. §§ 447.272, 447.321. Some states also receive CMS approval to make supplemental payments to hospitals and other providers under Section 1115 demonstration waivers. These

supplemental payments are governed by the terms and conditions of the individual demonstration waiver and may be subject to firm dollar limits and other requirements.

[21] States also maintain data that could be used to analyze per-enrollee spending, such as encounter data used by some states to develop managed care capitation rates. However, states' data are not suitable for purposes of examining spending across states as such data may not be fully comparable across states.

[22] State Medicaid agencies are required to submit the quarterly expenditure data by means of the Quarterly Medicaid Statement of Expenditures for the Medical Assistance Program, also known as the form CMS-64, within 30 days of the end of each quarter. 42 C.F.R. § 430.30. The data are stored in the Medicaid Budget and Expenditure System.

[23] States are required to have in operation a mechanized claims-processing and information-retrieval system based on certain federal requirements. *See* 42 U.S.C. § 1396b(r). For all claims filed on or after January 1, 1999, states have been required to electronically transmit claims data, including detailed individual enrollee encounter data, in a format consistent with MSIS. *See* 42 U.S.C. § 1396b(r)(1)(F).

[24] This project will result in a new data system known as Transformed–MSIS, or T-MSIS. The goals of T-MSIS include improving the timeliness, quality, and level of detail of the MSIS data and providing a link to the CMS-64 data in order to support improved program and financial management, evaluations, fraud identification, and program efficiency. T-MSIS data are not intended to replace the CMS-64 data. T-MSIS is scheduled to be implemented July 1, 2014. In September, 2013, the HHS Office of Inspector General reported that CMS had made some progress in implementing T-MSIS with 12 volunteer states, but raised concerns about the completeness and accuracy of T-MSIS data upon national implementation. See Department of Health and Human Services Office of Inspector General, *Early Outcomes Show Limited Progress for the Transformed Medicaid Statistical Information System*, OEI-05-12-00610 (Washington, D.C.: September 2013).

[25] For examples, see CMS, *2012 Actuarial Report on Financial Outlook for Medicaid* (Baltimore, Md.: 2012), and Medicaid and CHIP Payment and Access Commission (MACPAC), *March 2013 Report to the Congress on Medicaid and CHIP* (Washington, D.C.: March 15, 2013).

[26] These spending estimates include federal and state spending on regular Medicaid payments made to providers and managed care plans for covered services, as well as DSH and non-DSH supplemental payments, but do not include administrative costs. Enrollment is measured in terms of full-year-equivalent enrollees. Both enrollment and expenditure data include all enrollees, regardless of the scope of benefits offered.

[27] Adjustments are made by states to correct overpayments, underpayments, or reporting errors to spending reported in prior quarterly reports. Collections include reimbursement from private or public insurance plans or other third parties that are liable for some portion of enrollees' health care costs, as well as recoveries made through efforts to reduce waste, fraud, and abuse. The annual summary reports "roll up," or aggregate, the dollar amounts states reported in their quarterly reports for the year.

[28] This report is called the CMS-64 Base Financial Management Report. The other annual summary report that provides data on states' total spending by type of service is called the CMS-64 Net Services Financial Management Report.

[29] These sums may also include adjustments to spending for Medicaid expansion programs under the State Children's Health Insurance Program as well as for the traditional Medicaid program.

[30] In the other summary report, the CMS-64 Net Services Financial Management Report, the adjustments are applied to the current year's spending, by type of service, and program. For

example, if a state reported negative adjustments totaling $20 million to its spending on inpatient care services during the prior fiscal year, that $20 million would be subtracted from the state's current reported spending for that service, rather than being subtracted from its spending on inpatient care services for the prior year.

[31] As they do for adjustments, states must also submit a separate form to report collections but are not required to indicate the time period in which the original claims were paid.

[32] For California and the other five states (Alaska, Georgia, Indiana, Mississippi, and Utah), most of the difference is due to adjustments rather than collections. According to CMS officials, some states consistently report more adjustments than others.

[33] When states submit their quarterly CMS-64 expenditure reports, they must also submit an additional form or forms detailing any adjustments to spending reported for prior periods. In each form, the state indicates the amount of adjustment, positive or negative, by type of service, and the federal match that was claimed for that spending.

[34] The number of forms states must submit to report adjustments—and which would therefore need to be reviewed to manually apply adjustments to the appropriate time period—partly depends on the time period over which the original spending occurred. According to CMS officials, states report any adjustments to previously reported spending on separate forms by the quarter—or, in the case of spending from fiscal year 2008 or before, by the year—in which the spending was originally reported. For example, if a state needed to correct amounts reported throughout fiscal years 2009 and 2010, it would need to submit at least eight prior period adjustment forms—four for each year. The number of forms required also depends on whether the original spending was for the traditional Medicaid program operated under the Medicaid state plan, for programs operated under waivers, or both, because adjustments to spending for waiver programs must be reported separately for each waiver. CMS officials also told us that states report most adjustments within 2 years, but may report some adjustments, including those resulting from federal audits, 3 or more years after the original spending occurred. In such a case, adjusting a state's reported spending for a given year could involve compiling a dozen or more subsequent quarterly reports.

[35] In addition, while states were required to submit annual audits and reports on DSH payments in 2010, there are not similar reporting requirements for non-DSH supplemental payments. We have previously recommended that CMS take steps to improve states' reporting of supplemental payments and that Congress consider requiring CMS to take such steps. See GAO, *Medicaid: More Transparency of and Accountability for Supplemental Payments Are Needed,* GAO-13-48 (Washington, D.C.: Nov. 26, 2012).

[36] GAO, *Medicaid: States Reported Billions More in Supplemental Payments in Recent Years,* GAO-12-694 (Washington, D.C.: July 20, 2012).

[37] For example, some non-DSH supplemental payments to hospitals may be included with spending for inpatient or outpatient care. According to HHS officials, CMS has held training for states on completing the CMS-64 form and are continuing to work with states to help ensure accurate reporting of non-DSH supplemental payments on the CMS-64. Officials also noted that, in 2013, CMS began requiring states to annually submit data to demonstrate that Medicaid provider payments, including certain types of non-DSH supplemental payments, are below federal limits. CMS anticipates these submissions will assist the agency to identify errors in state reporting.

[38] Data from fiscal year 2013 suggest that many states that reported higher DSH payments reported lower non-DSH supplemental payments and vice versa.

[39] See Debra Lipson, Margaret Colby, Tim Lake, Su Liu, and Sarah Turchin, *Value for the Money Spent? Exploring the Relationship between Medicaid Costs and Quality* (Washington, D.C.:

Mathematica Policy Research, 2010), p. 6. Another argument for excluding these funds is that some states have used these payments to inappropriately increase federal Medicaid matching payments. See GAO, *High Risk Series: An Update*, GAO-11-278 (Washington, D.C.: February 2011), p. 163.

[40] On average, DSH payments represented about 4 percent of states' overall spending in fiscal year 2008, but that percentage varied significantly and, in three states (Louisiana, New Hampshire, and New Jersey), these payments represented more than 15 percent of overall spending. See table 3 in appendix IV and table 4 in appendix V for more detailed information about DSH payments in fiscal year 2008.

[41] This is the general approach that the Medicaid and CHIP Payment and Access Commission (MACPAC) used to distribute DSH payments among eligibility groups in its estimates of spending per enrollee. See Medicaid and CHIP Payment and Access Commission, *Report to the Congress on Medicaid and CHIP* (Washington, D.C.: June 2012), p. 138.

[42] In the CMS-64, spending for enrollees in capitated managed care plans is reported as payments to managed care organizations or prepaid health plans, not as payments for specific types of services.

[43] See *Medicaid Analytic eXtract* 2008 *Chartbook*, Table 3.2.

[44] Four states did not have reliable data available on the proportion of aged enrollees receiving long-term care services. Specifically, in Arizona, New Mexico and Wisconsin, more than 2 percent of all enrollees—and therefore likely a higher percentage of aged enrollees—received long-term care services through managed care plans and therefore were not represented in the FFS data used to identify enrollees who received long-term care services during the year. Maine was unable to accurately report its spending by service category. We also excluded a fifth state, Massachusetts, from this analysis because of errors in fiscal year 2008 CMS data.

[45] Our analysis of MSIS data showed that, on average, states spent $41,752 per enrollee for those receiving long-term care services in institutional settings in fiscal year 2008, compared to an average of $20,736 per enrollee for those receiving long-term care services in home- and community-based settings.

[46] See *Medicaid Analytic eXtract 2008 Chartbook*, Table A3.5. Four states did not have reliable data available on the proportion of enrollees receiving institutional care services. Specifically, in Arizona, New Mexico, and Wisconsin, more than 2 percent of all enrollees—and therefore likely a higher percentage of aged enrollees—received long-term care services through managed care plans and therefore were not represented in the FFS data used to identify enrollees who were ever institutionalized during the year. Maine was unable to accurately report its spending by service category.

[47] Our analysis of MSIS data showed that, for children who received services, states spent an average of about $8,056 per foster care child in fiscal year 2008 compared to an average of about $2,055 per non-foster-care child.

[48] One study found that, across all payers, per capita medical spending was $1,429 (about 42 percent) higher for obese people than for people of normal weight in 2006. The authors noted that costs attributable to obesity are due almost entirely to costs of treating diseases that obesity promotes, such as diabetes. See Eric A. Finkelstein, Justin G. Trogdon, Joel W. Cohen, and William Dietz, "Annual Medical Spending Attributable to Obesity: Payer- and Service-Specific Estimates," *Health Affairs*, 28, no. 5 (2009). The Congressional Budget Office found that annual per capita health care spending for current or former smokers was 11 to 16 percent higher than for people who have never smoked, depending on their ages, in

2008 dollars. See Congressional Budget Office, *Raising the Excise Tax on Cigarettes: Effects on Health and the Federal Budget* (Washington, D.C.: June 2012).

[49] See *Medicaid Analytic eXtract 2008 Chartbook*, Figure 2.10. These spending figures do not include DSH payments or other supplemental payments.

[50] See *Medicaid Analytic eXtract 2008 Chartbook* , Table A7.2.

[51] We did not assess differences among states in actual Medicaid FFS provider payment rates for specific services. To the extent that payment rates are driven by the costs of delivering health care services, differences across states in average wages for health care workers would translate into corresponding differences in payment rates. For more information on state Medicaid provider payment rates, see GAO, *Medicaid: Use of Claims Data for Analysis of Provider Payment Rates*, GAO-14-56R. (Washington, D.C.: Jan. 6, 2014.)

[52] See GAO-13-434, pp. 24-27. The most conservatively calculated health services cost index assumed that personnel accounted for 50 percent of the total cost to provide health services—the minimum proportion of costs attributed to personnel in Medicare's prospective payment systems for a variety of services. The differences among states were greater based on an index that assumed that personnel account for a higher percentage of total costs.

[53] Children in foster care, most of whom are eligible for Medicaid, are an especially vulnerable population because often they have been subjected to traumatic experiences involving abuse or neglect and they may suffer from multiple, serious mental health conditions. See GAO, *Children's Mental Health: Concerns Remain About Appropriate Services for Children in Medicaid and Foster Care*, GAO-13-15 (Washington, D.C.: Dec. 10, 2013).

[54] For example, encounter data may specify an enrollee's diagnosed health conditions or prescribed medications that may be used to infer such conditions.

[55] One consulting firm official told us that states with small populations in managed care may decide that the data and other challenges and costs involved with implementing risk adjustment outweigh the benefits.

[56] States initially base managed care rates on FFS data, but need to transition to encounter data after enrollees have been in managed care for several years because the FFS data become outdated.

[57] Some of the state and consulting firm officials told us that some managed care plans do not provide states with the complete or accurate encounter data that states are required to submit to CMS in MSIS. Some consulting firm officials suggested that states build incentives into their plan contracts to encourage plans to report accurate data. In addition, PPACA gives the Secretary of Health and Human Services the authority to withhold a state's federal Medicaid matching funds if the state does not report enrollee encounter data to MSIS, as required by HHS. 42 U.S.C. § 1396b(i)(25). A CMS official recently indicated that CMS has prioritized obtaining and validating states' encounter data in MSIS. In a prior report, we found that CMS planned to emphasize the need for more complete encounter data because the agency has determined that states' encounter data that do not include pricing information are not sufficient for setting rates. See GAO, *Medicaid Managed Care: CMS's Oversight of States' Rate Setting Needs Improvement*, GAO-10-810 (Washington, D.C.: Aug. 4, 2010).

[58] State officials told us that since the state transitions to risk adjustment may have resulted in plans receiving higher or lower payments, they have phased in risk-adjusted rate changes over several years to allow plans to adapt to potential payment changes.

[59] For more information on how economic changes may affect Medicaid enrollment, see GAO, *Medicaid: Prototype Formula Would Provide Automatic, Targeted Assistance to States*

during Economic Downturns. GAO-12-38, (Washington, D.C.: Nov. 10, 2011); and *Medicaid: Improving Responsiveness of Federal Assistance to States during Economic Downturns*. GAO-11-395 (Washington, D.C.: Mar. 31, 2011).

End Notes for Appendix I

[1] State Medicaid agencies are required to submit these aggregate expenditure data 30 days after a quarter has ended by means of the Quarterly Medicaid Statement of Expenditures for the Medical Assistance Program—also known as the form CMS-64 within the Medicaid Budget and Expenditure System. CMS uses the data to compute the federal financial participation for each state's Medicaid program costs. Federal Medicaid law requires states to make DSH payments to qualifying hospitals that serve large numbers of Medicaid and uninsured low-income patients. States also make other supplemental payments to hospitals and other providers that, for example, serve high-cost Medicaid enrollees.

[2] State Medicaid agencies are required to provide CMS, through MSIS, with quarterly electronic files approximately 45 days after a quarter has ended that contain data on the persons covered by Medicaid and on claims for medical services reimbursed by the Medicaid program.

[3] Adjustments are made to correct overpayments, underpayments, or reporting errors that relate to spending reported in prior quarterly reports. Collections include reimbursement from private or public insurance plans or other third parties that are liable for some portion of enrollees' health care costs, as well as recoveries made through efforts to reduce waste, fraud, and abuse.

[4] Specifically, we collapsed three eligibility groups (adults, unemployed adults, and enrollees who qualify for Medicaid under provisions of the Breast and Cervical Cancer Act) into the adult eligibility group, and three other eligibility groups (children, children of unemployed adults, and foster care children) into the children eligibility group.

[5] States were not required to separately report non-DSH supplemental payments until fiscal year 2010, and have not done so consistently since then. See GAO, *Medicaid: More Transparency and Accountability for Supplemental Payments Are Needed*, GAO-13-48 (Washington, D.C., Nov. 26, 2012).

[6] This is the general approach that the Medicaid and CHIP Payment and Access Commission (MACPAC) uses to distribute DSH payments among eligibility groups in its estimates of spending per enrollee. See Medicaid and CHIP Payment and Access Commission, *Report to the Congress on Medicaid and CHIP* (Washington, D.C.: June 2012), pp. 138-141.

End Notes for Appendix III

[1] In the other annual summary report, collections are reported as a separate line item, but adjustments are folded into the current year's spending, by type of service, and program.

[2] These sums may also include adjustments to spending for Medicaid expansion programs under the State Children's Health Insurance Program as well as for the traditional Medicaid program.

End Note for Appendix IV

[1] Under federal law, states may only claim federal matching funds for DSH payments made to qualifying hospitals up to the states' DSH allotments, which are based on a statutory formula and vary across the states. Individual hospitals may only receive DSH payments up to their hospital-specific limit. States also make DSH payments out of their allotment to institutions for mental disease and other mental health facilities that provide inpatient services. However, federal law limits the total amount of federal matching funds that states may claim for DSH payments made to these mental health facilities. 42 U.S.C. § 1396r-4.

In: Medicaid Spending by States
Editor: Hank Milford
ISBN: 978-1-63463-538-7

Chapter 2

MEDICAID FINANCING AND EXPENDITURES*

Alison Mitchell

SUMMARY

Medicaid is a means-tested entitlement program that finances the delivery of primary and acute medical services as well as long-term services and supports. Medicaid is a federal and state partnership that is jointly financed by both the federal government and the states.

The federal government's share for most Medicaid expenditures is called the federal medical assistance percentage (FMAP) rate. Generally determined annually, the FMAP formula is designed so that the federal government pays a larger portion of Medicaid costs in states with lower per capita incomes relative to the national average (and vice versa for states with higher per capita incomes). Federal Medicaid funding to states is open-ended.

The federal government provides states a good deal of flexibility in determining the composition of the state share (also referred to as the non-federal share) of Medicaid expenditures. As a result, there is significant variation from state to state in the funding sources used to finance the state share of Medicaid expenditures. In state FY2012, states reported that on average state general funds (i.e., revenues from personal income, sales, and corporate income taxes) made up 77% of the state share of Medicaid expenditures and the remaining 23% was financed by

* This is an edited, reformatted and augmented version of a Congressional Research Service publication R42640, prepared for Members and Committees of Congress, dated February 7, 2014.

"other state funds" (i.e., provider taxes, local government funds, and tobacco settlement funds).

In FY2012, Medicaid expenditures totaled $431 billion, with the federal government paying $249 billion, about 58% of the total. While Medicaid expenditures (like all health expenditures) generally grow at a rate faster than the economy, as measured by the gross domestic product (GDP), spending per enrollee under Medicaid tends to be lower than the per person spending for other forms of health insurance. One of the major factors impacting Medicaid spending is the economy. Also, state-specific factors, such as programmatic decisions and demographics, affect Medicaid expenditures and cause Medicaid spending to vary widely from state to state.

Starting in FY2014, Medicaid expenditures are expected to increase significantly as a result of the reforms enacted in the Patient Protection and Affordable Care Act (ACA, P.L. 111-148 as amended). The most noteworthy ACA change to Medicaid started January 1, 2014, when some states expanded Medicaid eligibility to adults under age 65 with income up to 133% of the federal poverty level (FPL) (effectively 138% FPL with the 5% FPL income disregard).

Following the June 28, 2012, Supreme Court decision in *National Federation of Independent Business v. Sebelius*, it is uncertain how many states will expand their Medicaid program to cover this new group. According to the Congressional Budget Office and the Joint Committee on Taxation, the expansion is expected to increase federal Medicaid expenditures by $612 billion from FY2014 to FY2022, which is $319 billion less than the estimate conducted prior to the Supreme Court decision.

This report provides an overview of Medicaid's financing structure, including both federal and state financing issues. The Medicaid expenditures section of the report discusses economic factors affecting Medicaid, state variability in spending, and projected program spending. Other issues that are examined include federal deficit reduction proposals affecting Medicaid and state fiscal conditions affecting Medicaid financing and services.

INTRODUCTION

Medicaid is a means-tested entitlement[1] program that finances the delivery of primary and acute medical services as well as long-term services and supports.[2] Medicaid is a federal and state partnership. The states are responsible for administering their Medicaid programs, and Medicaid is jointly financed by the federal government and the states. In FY2012, Medicaid is estimated to have provided health care services to 57 million individuals[3] at a total cost of $431 billion (including federal and state expenditures).[4]

Participation in Medicaid is voluntary, though all states, the District of Columbia, and the territories choose to participate. The federal government sets some basic requirements[5] for Medicaid, but states are provided flexibility to design their own version of Medicaid within the federal government's basic framework.

States incur Medicaid costs by making payments to service providers (e.g., for beneficiaries' doctor visits) and performing administrative activities (e.g., making eligibility determinations). The federal government reimburses states for a share of each dollar spent in accordance with their federally approved Medicaid state plans.

Medicaid is an entitlement for both states and individuals. The Medicaid entitlement to states ensures that, so long as states operate their programs within the federal requirements, states are entitled to federal Medicaid matching funds. This means that federal Medicaid spending is open-ended. Medicaid is also an individual entitlement, which means that anyone eligible for Medicaid under his or her state's eligibility standards is guaranteed Medicaid coverage.

This report provides an overview of Medicaid's financing structure including both federal and state financing issues. The Medicaid expenditures section of the report discusses economic factors affecting Medicaid, state variability in spending, and projected program spending. Other issues that are examined include congressional proposals to turn Medicaid into a block grant program, federal deficit reduction proposals affecting Medicaid, and state fiscal conditions affecting Medicaid financing and services.

MEDICAID FINANCING

The federal government and the states share the cost of Medicaid. The federal government reimburses states for a portion (i.e., the federal share) of each state's Medicaid program costs. Because federal Medicaid funding is an open-ended entitlement to states, there is no upper limit or cap on the amount of federal Medicaid funds a state may receive. In a typical year, the federal share of Medicaid expenditures is about 57%, which means the state share is about 43%.[6]

Federal Share

A primary goal of the federal Medicaid matching arrangement is to share the cost of providing health care services to low-income residents with the states. The Medicaid financing structure represents a clear fiscal commitment on the part of the federal government toward paying at least half (but not all) of the cost of Medicaid.[7]

The federal government's open-ended financial commitment to Medicaid provides a fiscal incentive for states to extend Medicaid coverage to more low-income individuals than a state might choose to fund without the federal Medicaid funding. However, this incentive is counterbalanced by the requirement for states to share in the cost of Medicaid.[8,9]

The Federal Medical Assistance Percentage (FMAP) Rate

The federal government's share of most Medicaid expenditures is established by the FMAP rate, which is generally determined annually and varies by state according to each state's per capita income relative to the U.S. per capita income.[10] The formula provides higher FMAP rates, or federal reimbursement rates, to states with lower per capita incomes and lower FMAP rates to states with higher per capita incomes. FMAP rates have a statutory minimum of 50% and a statutory maximum of 83%.[11] The formula for a given state is

$$FMAP_{state} = 1 - ((\text{Per capita income}_{state})^2/(\text{Per capita income}_{U.S.})^2 * 0.45)$$

The use of the 0.45 factor in the formula is designed to ensure that a state with per capita income equal to the U.S. average receives an FMAP rate of 55%, with a state share of 45%. In addition, the formula's squaring of per capita income provides higher FMAP rates to states with below-average per capita incomes than the states would otherwise receive (and vice versa).[12] In FY2014, FMAP rates range from 50% (15 states) to 73% (Mississippi).

Exceptions to the FMAP Rate and Open-Ended Funding

The FMAP rate is used to reimburse states for the federal share of most Medicaid expenditures, but exceptions to the regular FMAP rate have been made for certain states (e.g., the District of Columbia and the territories), situations (e.g., during economic downturns), populations (e.g., certain women with breast or cervical cancer and individuals in the Qualifying Individuals[13] program), providers (e.g., primary care physicians and Indian Health Service facilities), and services (e.g., family planning and home health services).[14] In addition, the federal share for most Medicaid administrative costs does not vary by state and is generally 50%.

While most federal Medicaid funding is provided on an open-ended basis, certain types of federal Medicaid funding are capped. For instance, federal disproportionate share hospital (DSH)[15] funding to states cannot exceed a state-specific annual allotment. Also, Medicaid programs in the territories (i.e., American Samoa, Guam, the Commonwealth of the Northern Mariana Islands, Puerto Rico, and the Virgin Islands) are subject to annual spending caps. Other exceptions to open-ended federal Medicaid funding include the Qualified Individuals program and waivers that allow states to operate outside of normal federal rules (which are subject to aggregate budget caps or cost-per-beneficiary caps).[16]

Medicaid and the Federal Budget Process

As discussed above, Medicaid is a federal entitlement to states, and in federal budget parlance entitlement spending is categorized as mandatory spending, which is also referred to as direct spending. However, Medicaid is an unusual mandatory spending program.

While most mandatory spending programs bypass the annual appropriations process and automatically receive funding each year according to either permanent or multi-year appropriations in the substantive law, Medicaid is funded in the annual appropriations acts. For this reason, Medicaid is referred to as an "appropriated entitlement."[17]

The level of spending for appropriated entitlements, like other entitlements, is based on the benefit and eligibility criteria established in law. The amount of budget authority provided in appropriations acts for Medicaid is based on budget projections for meeting the funding needs of the program. While most changes to the Medicaid program are made through statute, the fact that Medicaid is subject to annual appropriations process provides an opportunity for Congress to place funding limitations on specified activities in Medicaid, including the circumstances under which federal funds can be used to pay for abortions.

State Share

The federal government provides broad guidelines to states regarding allowable funding sources for the state share (also referred to as the non-federal share) of Medicaid expenditures. However, to a large extent, states are free to determine how to fund their share of Medicaid expenditures. As a result, there is significant variation from state to state in funding sources.

States can use state general funds (i.e., personal income, sales, and corporate income taxes) and "other state funds" (i.e., provider taxes, local government funds, tobacco settlement funds, etc.) to finance the state share of Medicaid.[18] Federal statute[19] allows as much as 60% of the state share to come from local government funding.[20] Federal regulations also stipulate that the state share not be funded with federal funds (Medicaid or otherwise).[21] In state fiscal year (SFY) 2012, on average, 77% of the state share of Medicaid expenditures was financed by state general funds, and the remaining 23% was financed by "other state funds."[22]

A few funding sources have received a great deal of attention over the past couple decades because states have used these funds in some financing mechanisms designed to maximize the amount of federal Medicaid funds coming to the state. This is referred to as "Medicaid maximization."[23] In general, some states have used "Medicaid maximization" strategies that involve the coordination of fund sources, such as provider taxes and intergovernmental transfers (IGTs), and payment policies, such as DSH and supplemental payments[24] to draw down federal Medicaid funds without expending much, if any, state general funds.

Provider Taxes

States are able to use revenues from health care provider taxes to help finance their share of Medicaid expenditures.[25] Federal statute and regulations define a provider tax as a health care-related fee, assessment, or other mandatory payment for which at least 85% of the burden of the tax revenue falls on health care providers.[26]

In order for states to be able to use the revenue generated from a provider tax to fund their state share of Medicaid expenditures, the provider tax must be both broad-based (i.e., imposed on all providers within a specified class of providers) and uniform (i.e., the same tax for all providers within a specified class of providers). Also, states are not allowed to hold the providers harmless for the cost of the provider tax (i.e., they cannot guarantee that providers receive their money back).

States first began using health care provider taxes, as well as provider donations,[27] to help finance the state share of Medicaid expenditures in the mid-1980s. In some cases, Medicaid providers initiated these provider tax and donation arrangements because states would often use the resulting revenue to increase Medicaid payment rates. Plus, these arrangements were often designed in such a way as to hold the Medicaid providers harmless for the cost of their taxes or donations (i.e., providers received their tax and donation money back through Medicaid rate increases).[28]

While not all states were using provider taxes to finance their share of Medicaid, some states were particularly aggressive in their use of provider taxes. As a result, in 1991, Congress passed the Medicaid Voluntary Contribution and Provider-Specific Tax Amendments (P.L. 102-234) to restrict the use of provider donations in financing Medicaid to extremely limited situations[29] and to limit states' ability to use provider tax revenue to qualify for federal Medicaid matching funds.

A number of states have approved additional provider taxes since the beginning of the most recent recession (December 2007 through June 2009),[30] despite federal statutory and regulatory limitations.[31] In SFY2013, 49 states and the District of Columbia used at least one provider tax to finance Medicaid.[32]

Provider taxes continue to cause tension between the federal government and the states. For this reason, some federal deficit reduction proposals recommend limiting states' ability to use provider taxes for Medicaid.[33]

Local Government Funds

As long as total local funds comprise less than 60% of the state share of Medicaid expenditures, local governments and local government providers can contribute to the state share of Medicaid payments through IGTs or certified public expenditures (CPEs). For IGTs, a local government transfers funds to the state government to be used to finance Medicaid. When CPEs are used to fund the state share, the local government certifies its Medicaid expenditures to the state, and then the state claims the federal Medicaid matching funds.[34]

Intergovernmental Transfers (IGTs)

IGTs are transfers of public funds between government entities, such as from counties to states or between state agencies. This financing mechanism is commonly used to enable states and local governments to carry out shared functions.

The federal government allows the use of IGTs in financing the state share of Medicaid expenditures.[35] In fact, some states require their counties to transfer certain local tax revenues to help fund the state share of Medicaid expenditures for certain government providers (e.g., community mental health centers or hospitals) located in these counties.[36] For example, New York requires counties to pay roughly 30% of the state share of Medicaid, which is 15% of total Medicaid expenditures for New York.[37]

IGTs are a legitimate state budget tool, but IGTs become problematic when they are used in financing schemes that draw down excess federal Medicaid matching funds without using much, if any, state general funds.[38] Specifically, some states use IGTs to fund supplemental payments in order to leverage federal Medicaid matching funds.

An example of this would be if a state Medicaid program made a $20 million supplemental payment to a local health care facility and then requested the federal Medicaid matching funds for the supplemental payment. With an FMAP rate of 50%, both the federal government and the state would fund $10 million of the supplemental payment. The point at which this type of financing mechanism becomes contentious is when some states have the local health care facility transfer back to the state most of the supplemental payment (e.g., $18 million of the $20 million payment) through an IGT. In this example, the local health care facility retains $2 million, the state nets $8 million to use for other Medicaid or non-Medicaid purposes, and the federal government paid $10 million.[39]

Certified Public Expenditures (CPEs)

CPEs are another way for states to use local government funds to finance the state share of Medicaid. Under a CPE, either state or local governmental entities, including government-owned providers (e.g., county hospitals or local education agencies) make Medicaid expenditures according to the state's approved Medicaid state plan. Then, the government entity certifies to the state Medicaid agency that the expenditures are eligible for federal Medicaid matching funds. Once the state receives this certification, the state can draw down the federal matching funds. Federal statute[40] specifies that the funds used to finance Medicaid through a CPE must be derived from state or local taxes.[41]

States employ CPEs differently. Some states use CPEs with local health department, and other states use CPEs with hospitals operated by state/local governments. CPEs are also commonly used for Medicaid services provided at schools. Specifically, local education agencies certify Medicaid expenditures for Medicaid school-based health care and related administrative services. Then, the state draws down the federal matching funds.[42]

Process for Federal Medicaid Funds Getting to States

States incur Medicaid costs by making payments to service providers (e.g., for beneficiaries' doctor visits) and performing administrative activities (e.g., making eligibility determinations). After a state has made Medicaid expenditures, it can draw down federal matching funds. The Medicaid financing structure is set up so that states can draw down federal Medicaid matching funds on a real time basis, and the federal government reconciles state Medicaid expenditures on a quarterly basis.[43]

The Centers for Medicare & Medicaid Services (CMS) makes quarterly grant awards to states to cover the federal share of Medicaid expenditures. The amount of each quarterly grant is determined on the basis of quarterly estimates submitted to CMS by each state's Medicaid agency on the Form CMS-37 at least 45 days before the beginning of each fiscal quarter.

After CMS analyzes states' estimates, states receive grant awards that authorize them to draw down federal funds as needed to pay the federal share of Medicaid expenditures. States draw down federal matching funds through commercial banks and the Federal Reserve System against a continuing letter of credit certified by the Secretary of the Treasury in favor of the state payee.[44]

Each state must submit a Form CMS 64 no later than 30 days after the end of each quarter with the state's accounting of actual recorded expenditures. CMS reviews the expenditures reported on the CMS-64 to reconcile the states' estimates from the CMS-37 with the actual documented expenditures to ensure that the reported expenditures are allowable under the Medicaid statute.

In order to qualify for federal Medicaid matching funds, state Medicaid expenditures must be allowable. If CMS is uncertain as to whether a particular state expenditure is allowable, then CMS must notify the state and provide an opportunity for a hearing. If the state does not comply, CMS may withhold payment or disallow claims for federal Medicaid matching funds until the issue has been resolved.[45]

MEDICAID EXPENDITURES[46]

Medicaid expenditures account for a significant portion of total health expenditures in the United States. While Medicaid expenditures (like all health expenditures) generally grow at a rate faster than the economy as measured by the gross domestic product (GDP), spending per enrollee under Medicaid tends to be lower than the per-enrollee spending for other forms of health insurance.

One of the major factors impacting Medicaid spending is the economy. Also, state-specific factors, such as policy decisions and demographics, impact Medicaid expenditures and cause Medicaid spending to vary widely from state to state. Estimating the growth of Medicaid expenditures is uncertain due to the Supreme Court decision in *National Federation of Independent Business v. Sebelius*.

Medicaid in Terms of National Health Expenditures

In calendar year 2012, Medicaid expenditures were 15% of all health expenditures in the United States, including acute care services, long-term services and supports, and administrative expenditures. Medicaid pays for a significant portion of all long-term services and supports. In 2010, Medicaid paid for 31% of all nursing facility and continuing care retirement community expenditures, 37% of all home health care expenditures, and 53% of all other health, residential, and personal care expenditures. Medicaid's share of national health expenditures for other services is relatively smaller, with Medicaid expenditures accounting for 18% of all hospital expenditures, 8% of all physician and clinical expenditures, and 7% of all dental expenditures.[47]

Trend in Medicaid Expenditures

The cost of Medicaid, like most health expenditures, has generally increased at a rate significantly faster than the overall rate of U.S. economic growth, as measured by GDP.[48] In the past, much of Medicaid's expenditure growth has been due to federal or state expansions of Medicaid eligibility criteria,[49] but per-enrollee costs for Medicaid have also increased faster than the economy. However, when compared to other forms of health insurance, Medicaid per-enrollee expenditures are relatively low.[50]

Figure 1 shows Medicaid expenditures from FY1997 to FY2012. These expenditures are broken down by the state expenditures, federal expenditures, and recession-related additional federal funding.

In FY2012, Medicaid spending on services and administrative activities in the 50 states, the District of Columbia, and the territories totaled $431 billion. Federal Medicaid expenditures totaled $249 billion, and state Medicaid expenditures were $182 billion, which was 42% of total Medicaid spending.[51] Medicaid FY2012 spending on services grew by the second-slowest rate since the program's inception due to the expiration of the recession-related additional federal funding, cost containment actions taking by states, and Medicaid enrollment growth slowing.[52]

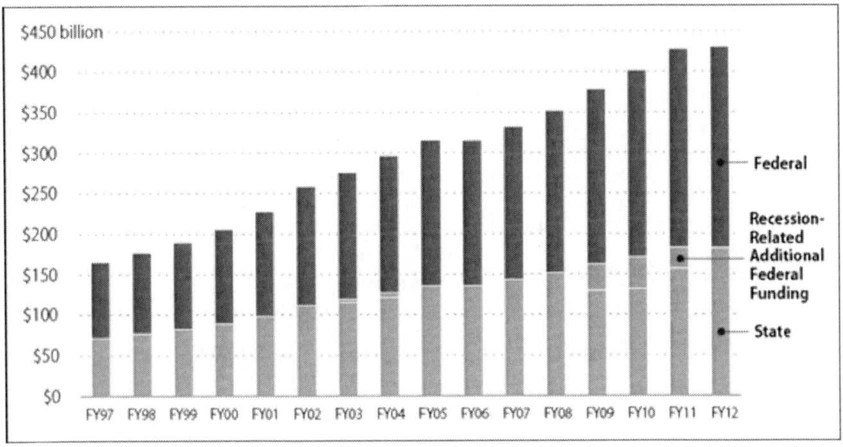

Source: Centers for Medicare & Medicaid, Form CMS-64 Data and Congressional Research Service communication with CMS.

Note: Recession-related additional federal Medicaid funding was provided in response to the 2001 recession and the 2007-2009 recession. For the 2001 recession, additional federal funding was provided through the Job Growth and Tax Relief Reconciliation Act of 2003 (P.L. 108-27). For the most recent recession, additional federal funding was provided through the American Recovery and Reinvestment Act of 2009 (ARRA, P.L. 111-5) and P.L. 111-226.

Figure 1. Federal and State Medicaid Expenditures. (FY1997 to FY2012; dollars in billions).

Per-Enrollee Medicaid Expenditures

Per-enrollee Medicaid expenditures averaged $6,982 in FY2011.[53] However, as shown in *Figure 2*, per-enrollee expenditures varied significantly by population group (i.e., children, adults, aged, and disabled) with the per-enrollee expenditures by population group ranging from $17,958 for disabled individuals to $2,851 for children.

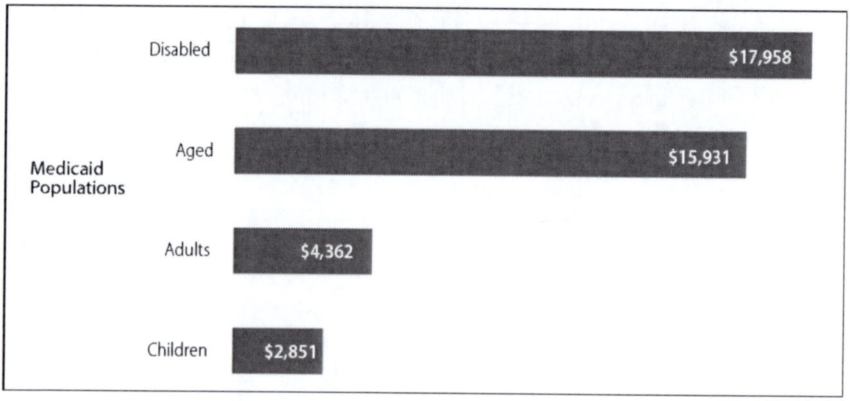

Figure 2. Expenditures Per Medicaid Enrollee by Major Population Groups. (FY2011).

One reason the aged and disabled populations have higher per-enrollee expenditures is because these populations consume most of the long-term services and supports, which comprise almost a quarter of all Medicaid expenditures (see *Figure 3*). Another reason for the difference in per-enrollee expenditures by population group is that children and adults tend to be healthier and therefore tend to have lower health care costs than the aged and disabled populations, even though a significant number of non-disabled adults are pregnant women.[54]

In FY2011, the aged and disabled populations together accounted for about 26% of Medicaid enrollment and 65% of Medicaid expenditures. In comparison, the children and adult populations accounted for about 74% of Medicaid enrollment and 35% of Medicaid expenditures.[55]

Medicaid Expenditures by Service Type

Figure 3 shows Medicaid expenditures by service type for FY2012. Long-term services and supports, which include nursing facility care and home- and community-based services, make up 26% of all Medicaid expenditures.[56] Managed care, which includes payments to managed care organizations,[57] primary care case management,[58] and non-comprehensive prepaid health plans,[59] accounts for 28% of total Medicaid expenditures. Hospitals receive 12% of total Medicaid expenditures in return for services provided to Medicaid fee-for-service[60] enrollees at the payment rates set by states.[61]

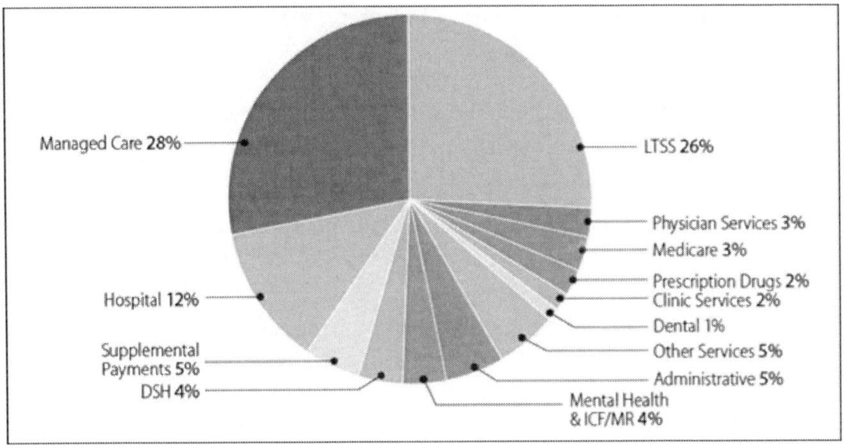

Source: CRS analysis of Centers for Medicare & Medicaid Services, Form CMS-64 Data.

Note: Prescription drug expenditures are net rebates. "Other services" include any expenditure type that amounts to less than 1% of total Medicaid expenditures, such as laboratory services, rural health, targeted case management, physical therapy, etc. LTSS comprise spending for nursing facility services, home health services, home- and community-based services, personal care services, etc. ICF/MR is an optional Medicaid benefit that enables states to provide comprehensive and individualized health care and rehabilitation services to individuals to promote their functional status and independence. Supplemental payments are Medicaid payments made to providers that are separate from and in addition to the standard payment rates for services rendered to Medicaid enrollees.

DSH: Disproportionate Share Hospital

ICF/MR: Intermediate Care Facility for individuals with Mental Retardation

LTSS: Long-Term Services and Supports

Figure 3. Total Medicaid Expenditures by Service Type. (FY2012).

Factors Affecting Medicaid Expenditures

Medicaid expenditures are influenced by economic, demographic, and programmatic factors. Economic factors include health care prices, unemployment rates, and individuals' wages. Demographic factors include population growth and the age distribution of the population. Programmatic factors include state decisions regarding optional eligibility groups, optional services, and provider payment rates. Other factors include the number of eligible individuals who enroll, utilization of covered services, and enrollment in other health insurance programs (including Medicare and private health insurance).[62]

The Economy

Medicaid enrollment is affected by economic factors, which in turn have an impact on Medicaid expenditures. Medicaid is referred to as a countercyclical program, which means Medicaid enrollment growth tends to accelerate when the economy weakens and to slow when the economy gains strength. During the most recent recession, researchers have estimated that for every 1% increase in the national unemployment rate, Medicaid enrollment increases by 1 million individuals.[63] People become eligible for Medicaid during economic downturns because they lose their job, have less income, or lose health benefits.[64]

Medicaid Enrollment

During and immediately after the 2007-2009 recession, growth in Medicaid expenditures was largely due to enrollment growth resulting from the higher unemployment rate.[65] The Bureau of Labor Statistics reported the seasonally adjusted national unemployment rate rose from 5.0% in December of 2007 to 9.5% in June of 2009, peaking at 10.0% in October 2010 (four months after the official end of the national recession).[66] Over roughly the same period, the estimated number of individuals ever enrolled[67] in Medicaid increased by 8.7%, from 58.8 million in FY2008 to an estimated 67.7 million in FY2010.[68] Medicaid enrollment growth occurred predominantly in the children and adult populations, while the Medicaid aged and disabled populations stayed relatively flat.[69]

Temporary FMAP Increase

As shown in **Figure 1**, the federal government covered the increase in total Medicaid expenditures from FY2009 through FY2011 through the temporary FMAP increase.[70] Federal Medicaid funding to states increased by $98.7 billion due to the temporary FMAP increase that was in place from October 1, 2008, through June 30, 2011. The temporary FMAP increase to states caused a shift in the federal and state shares of Medicaid expenditures, with the federal share of total Medicaid expenditures increasing from the typical 57% in FY2008 to 66% in FY2009, 67% in FY2010, 63% in FY2011, and decreasing back to 58% in FY2012.[71]

The temporary FMAP increase also caused shifts in the annual percent change in the federal and state Medicaid expenditures (*Figure 4*).

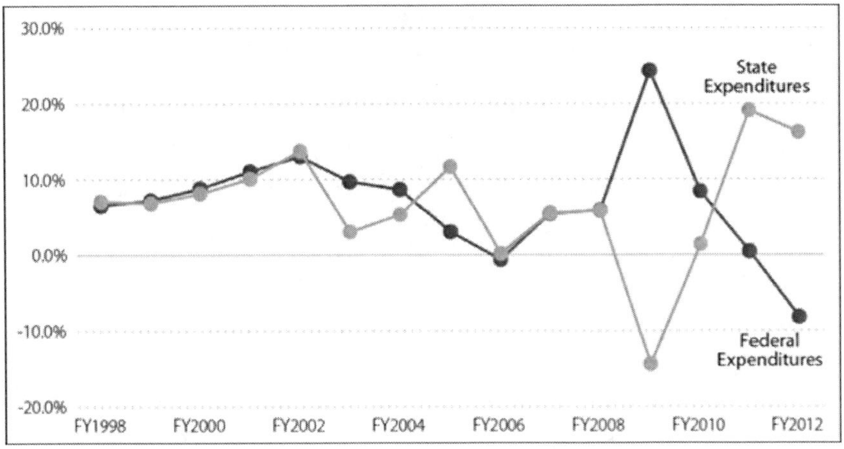

Source: Centers for Medicare & Medicaid Services, Form CMS-64 Data. Christopher J. Truffer, John D. Klemm, Christian J. Wolfe, et al., 2012 Actuarial Report on the Financial Outlook for Medicaid, Centers for Medicare & Medicaid Services' Office of the Actuary, 2013.

Figure 4. Annual Percent Change in Federal and State Medicaid Expenditures. (FY1998 to FY2012).

Prior to the 2001 recession, when additional federal funding was provided, federal and state Medicaid expenditures grew at the same rate. When additional federal funds were provided in FY2003 and FY2004, federal funds increased more than state funds. When the recession-related federal funds expired in FY2005, state expenditures increased more than federal Medicaid expenditures. In FY2006 through FY2008, federal and state Medicaid expenditures returned to increasing at the same rate. The temporary FMAP increase began October 1, 2008, causing federal Medicaid expenditures to increase significantly in FY2009 and FY2010 (24% and 8%, respectively), while state Medicaid expenditures decreased by 14% in FY2009 and were flat in FY2010. The temporary increase phased down beginning January 1, 2011, and expired June 30, 2011 (three-quarters of the way through FY2011), which caused state Medicaid expenditures to increase 19% in FY2011 while federal expenditures were relatively flat. In FY2012, state Medicaid expenditures increased 16% and federal Medicaid expenditures decreased by 8%.[72]

The shifts in the annual percent changes for federal and state Medicaid expenditures were more dramatic during the most recent recession because the federal government provided significantly more fiscal relief to states relative to the fiscal relief provided for the 2001 recession.

State Variability in Medicaid Spending

There is considerable variation in Medicaid spending from state to state. Some of the state variation is caused by demographic differences, such as state population and proportion of low-income residents. However, state variation in Medicaid per-enrollee expenditures is significant.

In order to participate in Medicaid, the federal government requires states to cover certain mandatory populations and benefits, but allows states to cover optional populations and services. In fact, an analysis of FY2001 Medicaid expenditures found that 61% of Medicaid expenditures are optional. Specifically, the analysis found that 39% of Medicaid expenditures were mandatory services for mandatory populations, while the remaining 61% of Medicaid expenditures were either optional services for mandatory groups (18%), mandatory services for optional groups (30%), or optional services for optional groups (12%).[73] Some of the sickest and poorest Medicaid enrollees are considered "optional," and many "optional benefits" provided under Medicaid often are integral health care services.[74]

State policy choices regarding optional populations and optional services cause variation in Medicaid spending. However, there are other reasons Medicaid spending varies from state to state.

Some of the state variation in Medicaid per-enrollee expenditures is due to differences across states in the demographics of Medicaid enrollees. For instance, states with lower-than-average proportions of elderly and disabled Medicaid enrollees and higher-than-average proportions of Medicaid enrollees who are low-income children and adults would be expected to have lower than average per-enrollee Medicaid expenditures.[75]

State variation in Medicaid per-enrollee expenditures is also due to variation in utilization and provider payment rates.[76] One analysis of disabled Medicaid enrollees found that utilization accounted for a significant amount of the variation in per-enrollee Medicaid expenditures. Specifically, the variation was attributed to utilization of inpatient hospital services and prescription drugs. The study found little difference in the per-enrollee Medicaid expenditures for ambulatory visits, such as physician, outpatient hospital, and clinic services.[77]

Projected Medicaid Expenditures

Over the next 10 years, Medicaid expenditures are projected to increase significantly, mainly due to the changes enacted by the Patient Protection and

Affordable Care Act (ACA, P.L. 111-148 as amended), with the Medicaid provisions in ACA representing the most considerable federal legislative change to Medicaid since its enactment in 1965.

ACA Medicaid Expansion

The most noteworthy ACA change to Medicaid is the expansion of Medicaid eligibility to adults under age 65 with income up to 133% of the federal poverty level (FPL) (effectively 138% FPL with the 5% FPL income disregard).[78] Originally, the assumption was that all states would implement the ACA Medicaid expansion in 2014 as required in statute because implementing the ACA Medicaid expansion was required in order for states to receive *any* federal Medicaid funding. However, on June 28, 2012, the United States Supreme Court issued its decision in *National Federation of Independent Business v. Sebelius*, finding that the federal government cannot terminate the federal Medicaid funding states are receiving for their current Medicaid program if a state refuses to implement the ACA Medicaid expansion.

Since the federal government cannot terminate current Medicaid federal matching funds if a state refuses to implement the Medicaid expansion required by the ACA, the Supreme Court's ruling in *NFIB* effectively made state participation in the ACA Medicaid expansion voluntary. On January 1, 2014, 24 states and the District of Columbia implemented the ACA Medicaid expansion, and Michigan is planning to implement the expansion on April 1, 2014.[79] Among the remaining states, some states (e.g., New Hampshire, Utah, and Virginia) are expected to debate the ACA Medicaid expansion issue during this year's legislative session.[80]

Prior to the Supreme Court decision, when it was assumed all states would implement the ACA Medicaid expansion, the Congressional Budget Office (CBO) and the Joint Committee on Taxation (JCT) estimated that the ACA Medicaid expansion would increase Medicaid and the State Children's Health Insurance Program (CHIP) enrollment by 13 million in FY2014 increasing to 17 million by FY2022, which CBO estimated would increase federal Medicaid expenditures by $931 billion from FY2012 to FY2022.[81]

According to the updated estimate, in each year between FY2014 and FY2022, the number of individuals covered by the ACA Medicaid expansion will be 3 million to 5 million less than estimated before the Supreme Court decision.[82] Specifically, CBO estimates the ACA Medicaid expansion will increase Medicaid and CHIP enrollment by 8 million in FY2014 increasing to 13 million by FY2020.[83] As shown in Figure 5, from FY2014 to FY2022, federal Medicaid expenditures resulting from the ACA health insurance coverage provisions (including the ACA Medicaid expansion) are estimated to be $610 billion, which is $321 billion less than the cost estimated conducted prior to the Supreme Court's decision. [84]

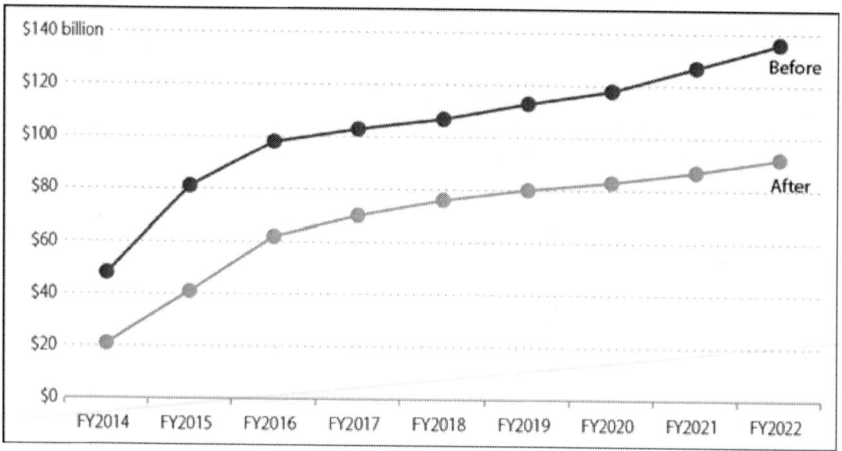

Source: Congressional Budget Office, Estimates for the Insurance Coverage Provisions of the Affordable Care Act Updated for the Recent Supreme Court Decision, July 2012; Congressional Budget Office, The Budget and Economic Outlook: 2014 to 2024, February 2014.

Note: Figure represents outlays in Medicaid only. CBO and JCT estimates that lower projected Medicaid spending due to some states not implementing the ACA Medicaid expansion would be offset by increased spending for the ACA insurance coverage provisions.

Figure 5. Estimated Federal Medicaid and CHIP Outlays for the ACA Medicaid Expansion Before and After the Supreme Court Decision. (FY2014 to FY2022; dollars in billions).

Other ACA Provisions

ACA makes a number of other changes to the Medicaid program that are expected to impact Medicaid expenditures.[85] Some ACA provisions that are expected to increase Medicaid expenditures include payments to the territories, the new Community First Choice Option,[86] the removal of barriers to providing home- and community-based services, and the extension of the Money Follows the Person demonstration.[87] Other provisions in ACA are expected to reduce Medicaid expenditures, including changes to prescription drug coverage and DSH payments.[88]

CURRENT ISSUES

Federal Deficit Reduction

Federal Medicaid expenditures account for almost 8% of all federal spending.[89] As a result, controlling federal Medicaid spending has been a focus of deficit reduction and budget proposals, such as the National Commission on Fiscal Responsibility and Reform's final report, the Bipartisan Policy Center's Debt Reduction Task Force proposal, the President's FY2014 budget, and the House FY2014 Budget Resolution.

The National Commission on Fiscal Responsibility and Reform's final report included savings from Medicaid totaling $58 billion over 10 years. The provisions with Medicaid savings included eliminating states' ability to fund Medicaid through provider taxes and covering dual eligible beneficiaries under managed care arrangements.[90]

The Bipartisan Policy Center's Debt Reduction Task Force estimated its proposals would reduce federal Medicaid expenditures by about $25 billion over 10 years. The task force proposed removing barriers for states to use managed care to cover dual eligible beneficiaries and limiting the growth in Medicaid expenditures by changing the structure of Medicaid financing.[91]

The President's FY2014 budget included a number of Medicaid provisions estimated by the Administration to reduce federal Medicaid expenditures by $22 billion over the next 10 years. The Medicaid provisions in the President's budget included limiting Medicaid reimbursement of durable medical equipment, "rebasing" Medicaid DSH payments, and prescription drug changes.[92]

The House FY2014 Budget Resolution (H.Con.Res. 25), based on Representative Ryan's *Path to Prosperity: A Responsible Balanced Budget* document, proposed making two significant programmatic changes to the Medicaid program. The proposal would repeal certain Medicaid provisions in ACA and convert Medicaid into a block grant program. In addition to these programmatic changes, the budget proposal suggests significant reductions to the federal Medicaid funding. Together these provisions are estimated to reduce federal Medicaid expenditures by $1.4 trillion over 10 years.

State Fiscal Conditions

During periods of economic downturn, state Medicaid programs face dual pressures. First, program enrollment increases at a faster rate when job and income losses lead more people to become eligible for Medicaid. Second, it can be more difficult to finance the state share of Medicaid costs because state revenue growth generally weakens during economic downturns.

When viewed nationally, Medicaid is the largest or second-largest item in state budgets depending on how it is measured. In terms of *total* state spending (i.e., funds from all state and federal sources), in SFY 2012, Medicaid was the largest component of the budget at an estimated 24% of *total* state spending. However, Medicaid is the second-largest component in terms of state *general fund* spending (i.e., the portion that states must finance on their own through taxes and other means). In SFY2012, Medicaid expenditures were an estimated 19% of state general fund spending, while elementary and secondary education spending was 35%.[93]

Throughout the recession, Medicaid expenditures grew as a percent of total state spending and shrank as a percent of state general fund spending because the federal government absorbed most of the recession-related increase in Medicaid expenditures through the temporary increase to FMAP rates.[94] However, with the phaseout of the temporary increase to FMAP rates in SFY2011, Medicaid expenditures as a share of state general fund spending grew from 15.8% in SFY2010 to an estimated 19% in SFY2012.[95]

While total Medicaid spending (i.e., including both federal and state spending) grew throughout the recession, total state tax revenues are estimated to have declined by 10.2% from the fourth quarter of 2007 to the fourth quarter of 2009.[96] Even with the temporary increase to FMAP rates moderating the impact of Medicaid expenditure growth on state general fund spending, many states faced budget deficits. A study from the Government Accountability Office notes that while these fiscal tensions existed for nearly all states during the economic downturn, any given state's capacity to finance the state share of Medicaid costs differed based on variables such as the state's economic condition, revenue structure, Medicaid program design, etc. Moreover, among states, economic downturns varied widely in their onset, depth, and duration, and generally do not coincide exactly with national recessions.[97]

Even though the national recession officially ended in June 2009, state tax revenues did not start increasing until the first fiscal quarter of 2010. States have experienced 14 consecutive quarters of revenue growth, but states are expecting a softening in revenue collections for SFY2014, with states projecting revenues to rise by only 0.8%.[98] Due to the fiscal pressure from the recession, nearly every state focused on Medicaid cost containment, and this focus is expected to continue in SFY2014 with the expected softening of state revenues.[99]

Because states had been prohibited from curbing the cost of Medicaid by restricting eligibility standards due to the maintenance of effort (MOE) requirements initially enacted under ARRA and later expanded and extended under ACA,[100] over the past few years, states have focused cost containment strategies on reducing provider rates, making changes to their benefit packages, or implementing limitations on the use of benefits.[101] However, with the exception of eligibility standards for children, states now (as of January 1, 2014) have the ability to reduce the cost of Medicaid through reductions to Medicaid eligibility standards. Eleven states (Illinois, Indiana, Louisiana, Maine, Minnesota, New Mexico, New York, Oklahoma, Rhode Island, Vermont, and Wisconsin) reported plans to tighten eligibility for their adult population groups in 2014.[102]

Due to Medicaid's federal/state financing structure, for states to generate $1 of savings in the state share of Medicaid spending, they would have to reduce their overall Medicaid spending by $2 to almost $4, depending on each state's regular FMAP rate. For example, in a state with a FMAP rate of 50%, to obtain state-share savings in the amount of $20 million the state would have to reduce total federal and state Medicaid spending by approximately $40 million. In a state with a FMAP rate of 65%, to obtain state-share savings in the amount of $20 million the state would have to reduce total federal and state share Medicaid spending by approximately $57 million. The degree to which a state is willing to cut the state share of its Medicaid spending might depend in part on the loss of federal dollars it would also face as a result of these reductions. This issue is a larger issue for states with higher FMAP rates, which have to cut their Medicaid program significantly to find small amounts of savings in state share.[103]

The softening of revenue collections only conveys part of the fiscal challenges for states because the reported gaps do not reflect the underfunding of pensions and retiree health care liabilities. Also, in recent years, budget gaps have sometimes been reduced temporarily by nonrecurring resources, such as rainy day funds.[104]

Prior to the recession, Medicaid was a fiscal challenge for states because Medicaid spending was growing faster than state revenues. This problem continued through the recession, and the trend is expected to continue for the foreseeable future.[105]

The Centers for Medicare & Medicaid Services' Office of the Actuary recently estimates Medicaid expenditures will increase by an average annual amount of 6.4% from FY2012 through FY2021.[106] At this rate of growth, Medicaid expenditure growth would significantly outpace historic growth rates for state revenues.[107] Thus, while the fiscal environment for states is improving, states continue to face challenges with the ongoing costs of Medicaid and the potential future costs of the ACA Medicaid expansion.[108]

End Notes

1 Entitlement means that individuals who meet state eligibility requirements, which must also meet federal minimum requirements, are entitled to Medicaid coverage.

2 For more information about the Medicaid program, see CRS Report R43357, Medicaid: An Overview, coordinated by Alison Mitchell.

3 This enrollment figure is measured according to "person-year equivalents," which is the average enrollment over the course of a year. Christopher J. Truffer, John D. Klemm, Christian J. Wolfe, et al., 2012 Actuarial Report on the Financial Outlook for Medicaid, Centers for Medicare & Medicaid Services' Office of the Actuary, 2013.

4 U.S. Department of Health and Human Services, Centers for Medicare and Medicaid Services, Form CMS-64 data.

5 The federal government requires states cover certain populations and benefits. On June 28, 2012, the United States Supreme Court issued its decision in National Federation of Independent Business v. Sebelius, finding that the federal government cannot terminate current Medicaid program federal matching funds if a state refuses to implement the Medicaid expansion required by the Patient Protection and Affordable Care Act (ACA, P.L. 111-148), which expands Medicaid eligibility to include non-elderly, non-pregnant adults under 133% of the federal poverty level. If a state accepts the new ACA Medicaid expansion funds, it must abide by the new expansion coverage rules, but, based on the Court's opinion, it appears that a state can refuse to participate in the expansion without losing any of its current federal Medicaid matching funds.

6 For FY2009 through FY2011, the federal share of Medicaid expenditures was higher than usual due to the temporary FMAP increase provided to states from October 1, 2008, through June 30, 2011. The temporary FMAP increase was originally provided through the American Recovery and Reinvestment Act of 2009 (P.L. 111-5) and extended through P.L. 111-226.

7 Andy Schneider and David Rousseau, The Medicaid Resource Book, The Kaiser Commission on Medicaid and the Uninsured, Publication Number 2236, January 17, 2003; Teresa A. Coughlin and Stephen Zuckerman, States' Use of Medicaid Maximization Strategies to Tap Federal Revenues: Program Implications and Consequences, The Urban Institute, June 2002.

8 Ibid.

[9] State decisions regarding Medicaid eligibility levels are determined based on a number of state-specific factors, including policy decisions about which optional eligibility groups should receive Medicaid coverage.

[10] For more detail about FMAP, see CRS Report R42941, Medicaid's Federal Medical Assistance Percentage (FMAP), FY2014, by Alison Mitchell and Evelyne P. Baumrucker.

[11] Section 1905(b) of the Social Security Act.

[12] For example, assume that U.S. per capita income is $40,000. In state A with a below-average per capita income of $38,000, the FMAP formula produces an FMAP rate of 59.39%; if the formula did not include a squaring of per capita income, it would instead produce a lower FMAP rate of 57.25%. In state B with an above-average per capita income of $42,000, the FMAP formula produces an FMAP rate of 50.39%; if the formula did not include a squaring of per capita income, it would instead produce a higher FMAP rate of 52.75%.

[13] States are required to pay Medicare Part B premiums for Medicare beneficiaries with income between 120% and 135% FPL and limited assets (referred to as "qualifying individuals"), up to a specified dollar allotment.

[14] For more detail about the FMAP exceptions, see CRS Report R42941, Medicaid's Federal Medical Assistance Percentage (FMAP), FY2014, by Alison Mitchell and Evelyne P. Baumrucker.

[15] The federal Medicaid statute requires that states make disproportionate share (DSH) adjustments to the payment rates of hospitals treating large numbers of low-income and Medicaid patients. For more information about Medicaid DSH payments, see CRS Report R42865, Medicaid Disproportionate Share Hospital Payments, by Alison Mitchell.

[16] In addition, some states have chosen to expand their Medicaid programs using capped federal allotments for the State Children's Health Insurance Program (CHIP). However, this does not affect the open-ended nature of federal funding for Medicaid. Once these states have exhausted their CHIP allotments, they revert to using Medicaid funds. For more information about CHIP, see CRS Report R40444, State Children's Health Insurance Program (CHIP): A Brief Overview, by Elicia J. Herz and Evelyne P. Baumrucker.

[17] For more information about "appropriated entitlements," see CRS Report RS20129, Entitlements and Appropriated Entitlements in the Federal Budget Process, by Bill Heniff Jr.

[18] Ibid.

[19] Section 1902(a)(2) of the Social Security Act.

[20] The federal statute allows for the significant use of local funds in financing Medicaid because local governments financed a significant amount of the health care services provided to low-income individuals prior to the enactment of Medicaid. The Patient Protection and Affordable Care Act (ACA, P.L. 111-148) included a provision that restricts states from increasing required local contributions to the state share of Medicaid. Specifically, in the case of a state that requires a political subdivision within the state to contribute to the non-federal share of expenditures, such state would not be eligible for an increase in its FMAP rate (under ACA or the American Recovery and Reinvestment Act of 2009, P.L. 111-5) if the state requires that political subdivisions pay a greater percentage of the non-federal share of expenditures (including expenditures for DSH payments) than amounts that would have been required as of December 31, 2009. Voluntary contributions are not considered "required" contributions. (Medicaid and CHIP Payment and Access Commission, Report to the Congress on Medicaid and CHIP, March 2012.)

[21] 42 C.F.R. 433.51(c).

[22] National Association of State Budget Officers, Fiscal Year 2010 State Expenditure Report: Examining Fiscal 2011- 2013 State Spending, 2013.

[23] National Health Policy Forum at The George Washington University, The Basics: Medicaid Financing, February 4, 2011; U.S. Government Accountability Office, Medicaid Financing: Long-Standing Concerns about Inappropriate State Arrangements Support Need for Improved Federal Oversight, testimony of Marjorie Kanof before U.S. Congress, House of Representatives, Committee on Oversight and Government Reform, GAO-08-255T, November 1, 2007; Andy Schneider and David Rousseau, The Medicaid Resource Book, The Kaiser Commission on Medicaid and the Uninsured, Publication Number 2236, January 17, 2003; Teresa A. Coughlin and Stephen Zuckerman, States' Use of Medicaid Maximization Strategies to Tap Federal Revenues: Program Implications and Consequences, The Urban Institute, June 2002.

[24] Supplemental payments are Medicaid payments made to providers that are separate from and in addition to the standard payment rates for services rendered to Medicaid enrollees. Often, providers receive supplemental payments in a lump sum.

[25] For more information about Medicaid provider taxes, see CRS Report RS22843, Medicaid Provider Taxes, by Alison Mitchell.

[26] The statute regarding provider taxes can be found in Section 1903(w) of the Social Security Act, and the accompanying regulations can be found at 42 C.F.R. 433.

[27] Provider donations are any donation or other voluntary payment made to a state or unit of local government by a health care provider. Section 1903(w)(2) of the Social Security Act.

[28] Andy Schneider, Risa Elias, Rachel Garfield, David Rousseau, and Victoria Wachino, The Medicaid Resource Book, Kaiser Commission on Medicaid and the Uninsured, July 2002.

[29] Provider donations are permissible if they do not exceed $5,000 per year in the case of an individual provider or $50,000 per year in the case of a "health care organization entity" (42 C.F.R. 433.66(a)(1)). Also, provider donations are allowed if the donations are made by a hospital, clinic, or similar entity (such as federally qualified health centers) for the direct costs of state or local agency personnel who are stationed at the facility to determine the eligibility of individuals for Medicaid or to provide outreach services to eligible (or potentially eligible) Medicaid individuals (i.e., outstationed eligibility workers) (42 C.F.R. 433.66(a)(2)). Provider donations for outstationed eligibility workers may not exceed 10% of a state's administrative costs for the Medicaid program (42 C.F.R. 433.67).

[30] Recession dates are designated by the National Bureau of Economic Research (NBER).

[31] The National Governors Association and the National Association of State Budget Officers, The Fiscal Survey of States, various years.

[32] Vernon K. Smith, Robin Rudowitz, and Laura Snyder, Medicaid in a Historic Time of Transformation: Results from a 50-State Medicaid Budget Survey for State Fiscal Years 2013 and 2014, Kaiser Commission on Medicaid and the Uninsured, October 2013.

[33] Department of Health and Human Services, Fiscal Year 2013 Budget in Brief: Strengthening Health and Opportunity for All Americans, February 2012; The National Commission on Fiscal Responsibility and Reform, The Moment of Truth, December 2010; Congressional Budget Office, Budget Options Volume I: Health Care, December 2008.

[34] U.S. Government Accountability Office, Medicaid: CMS Needs More Information on the Billions of Dollars Spent on Supplemental Payments, GAO-08-614, May 2008.

[35] Section 1903(w)(6) of the Social Security Act. 42 CFR 433.51.

[36] U.S. Government Accountability Office, Medicaid: CMS Needs More Information on the Billions of Dollars Spent on Supplemental Payments, GAO-08-614, May 2008.; National Health Policy Forum at The George Washington University, The Basics: Medicaid

Financing, February 4, 2011; Medicaid and CHIP Payment and Access Commission, Report to the Congress on Medicaid and CHIP, March 2012.

[37] Michael Birnbaum, Medicaid in New York: Current Roles, Recent Experience, and Implications of Federal Reform, Medicaid Institute at United Hospital Fund, December 2010.

[38] U.S. General Accounting Office, Medicaid: Intergovernmental Transfers Have Facilitated State Financing Schemes, GAO-04-574T, March 18, 2004; National Health Policy Forum at The George Washington University, The Basics: Medicaid Financing, February 4, 2011; Teresa A. Coughlin and Stephen Zuckerman, States' Use of Medicaid Maximization Strategies to Tap Federal Revenues: Program Implications and Consequences, The Urban Institute, June 2002.

[39] U.S. Government Accountability Office, Medicaid Financing: Federal Oversight Initiative Is Consistent with Medicaid Payment Principles but Needs Greater Oversight, GAO-07-214, March 2007.; U.S. General Accounting Office, Medicaid: Intergovernmental Transfers Have Facilitated State Financing Schemes, GAO-04-574T, March 18, 2004; Teresa A. Coughlin and Stephen Zuckerman, States' Use of Medicaid Maximization Strategies to Tap Federal Revenues: Program Implications and Consequences, The Urban Institute, June 2002.

[40] Section 1903(w)(6) of the Social Security Act. 42 CFR 433.51.

[41] Medicaid and CHIP Payment and Access Commission , Report to the Congress on Medicaid and CHIP, March 2012.

[42] Ibid.

[43] 42 C.F.R. 430.30.

[44] Ibid.

[45] 42 C.F.R. 430.35 and 42 C.F.R. 430.42

[46] Data in this section are provided for different years (i.e., FY2011, FY2010, or calendar year 2010) because Medicaid data are collected from states at different times for different purposes. For each type of expenditure, the most recent data are provided.

[47] Centers for Medicare & Medicaid Services, National Health Expenditures Data.

[48] Christopher J. Truffer, John D. Klemm, Christian J. Wolfe, et al., 2012 Actuarial Report on the Financial Outlook for Medicaid, Centers for Medicare & Medicaid Services' Office of the Actuary, 2013.

[49] Rachel Garfield, Lisa Clemans-Cope, Emily Lawton, et al., Enrollment-Driven Expenditure Growth: Medicaid Spending during the Economic Downturn, FFY2007-2010, Kaiser Commission on Medicaid and the Uninsured, Publication #8309, May 2012.

[50] Christopher J. Truffer, John D. Klemm, Christian J. Wolfe, et al., 2011 Actuarial Report on the Financial Outlook for Medicaid, Centers for Medicare & Medicaid Services' Office of the Actuary, March 2012.

[51] U.S. Department of Health and Human Services, Centers for Medicare and Medicaid Services, Form CMS-64 data.

[52] Christopher J. Truffer, John D. Klemm, Christian J. Wolfe, et al., 2012 Actuarial Report on the Financial Outlook for Medicaid, Centers for Medicare & Medicaid Services' Office of the Actuary, 2013.

[53] This figure excludes Medicaid expenditures for DSH, the territories, and administrative costs. Also, this figure is based on Medicaid enrollment measured by person-year equivalents, which is the average enrollment over the course of a year. Christopher J. Truffer, John D. Klemm, Christian J. Wolfe, et al., 2012 Actuarial Report on the Financial Outlook for Medicaid, Centers for Medicare & Medicaid Services' Office of the Actuary, 2013.

[54] Ibid; Andy Schneider and David Rousseau, The Medicaid Resource Book, The Kaiser Commission on Medicaid and the Uninsured, Publication Number 2236, January 17, 2003.

[55] Christopher J. Truffer, John D. Klemm, Christian J. Wolfe, et al., 2012 Actuarial Report on the Financial Outlook for Medicaid, Centers for Medicare & Medicaid Services' Office of the Actuary, 2013.

[56] For more information about long-term services and supports, see CRS Report R43328, Medicaid Coverage of Long-Term Services and Supports, by Kirsten J. Colello.

[57] States contract with managed care organizations to provide a comprehensive package of benefits to enrolled Medicaid beneficiaries, primarily on a capitated basis (i.e., a set amount per enrollee regardless of the services utilized).

[58] Under primary care case management, states contract with primary care physicians to provide case management services to Medicaid enrollees. For these enrollees, other services are generally provided on a fee-for-service basis.

[59] States contract with health plans to provide non-comprehensive benefits (e.g., inpatient behavioral health care or dental care).

[60] There are two major types of service payment systems under Medicaid—fee-for-service (FFS) and managed care. The FFS system was the predominant system of care both within and outside of Medicaid until about the mid-1990s. Under FFS, beneficiaries have unrestricted provider choice; that is, they can seek services from any Medicaid participating provider. Hence, beneficiaries are largely responsible for their own medical care management and coordination. Under managed care, states purchase or establish a network of providers for their Medicaid enrollees through contracts with health plans and/or providers who agree to accept Medicaid patients and to meet certain requirements to ensure timely access to care.

[61] Hospitals also receive a significant portion of both the Medicaid DSH funding and the supplemental payments.

[62] Christopher J. Truffer, John D. Klemm, Christian J. Wolfe, et al., 2011 Actuarial Report on the Financial Outlook for Medicaid, Centers for Medicare & Medicaid Services' Office of the Actuary, March 2012; Andy Schneider and David Rousseau, The Medicaid Resource Book, The Kaiser Commission on Medicaid and the Uninsured, Publication Number 2236, January 17, 2003.

[63] John Holahan and A. Bowen Garrett, Rising Unemployment, Medicaid and the Uninsured, Kaiser Commission on Medicaid and the Uninsured, Publication #7850, January 2009.

[64] Rachel Garfield, Lisa Clemans-Cope, Emily Lawton, et al., Enrollment-Driven Expenditure Growth: Medicaid Spending during the Economic Downturn, FFY2007-2010, Kaiser Commission on Medicaid and the Uninsured, Publication #8309, May 2012.

[65] John Holahan, Lisa Clemans-Cope, Emily Lawton, et al., Medicaid Spending Growth of the Last Decade and the Great Recession, 2000-2009, Kaiser Commission on Medicaid and the Uninsured, Publication 8152, February 2011; Rachel Garfield, Lisa Clemans-Cope, Emily Lawton, et al., Enrollment-Driven Expenditure Growth: Medicaid Spending during the Economic Downturn, FFY2007-2010, Kaiser Commission on Medicaid and the Uninsured, Publication #8309, May 2012.

[66] Bureau of Labor Statistics, Labor Force Statistics from the Current Population Survey, available at http://data.bls.gov/pdq/SurveyOutputServlet?data_tool=latest_numbers& series _id=LNS14000000.

[67] Since there is a lot of turnover in the Medicaid program, Medicaid enrollment measured in different ways can produce vastly different enrollment figures. Medicaid enrollment could be measured by "ever enrolled" persons (i.e., the number of people covered by Medicaid for any period of time during the year), "person-year equivalents" (i.e., the average enrollment

over the course of the year), and "point-in-time" (i.e., the number of Medicaid enrollees at a specified date). The annual count of Medicaid enrollees measured by "ever enrolled" persons will always exceed Medicaid enrollment measured by "person-year equivalents."

68 MACPAC, March 2011 Report to the Congress on Medicaid and CHIP, Table 2, March 2011. Federal fiscal year 2008 ran from October 1, 2007, through September 30, 2008, and federal fiscal year 2010 ran from October 1, 2009, through September 30, 2010.

69 John Holahan, Lisa Clemans-Cope, Emily Lawton, et al., Medicaid Spending Growth of the Last Decade and the Great Recession, 2000-2009, Kaiser Commission on Medicaid and the Uninsured, Publication 8152, February 2011.

70 The temporary FMAP increase was originally provided through the American Recovery and Reinvestment Act of 2009 (ARRA, P.L. 111-5) for nine fiscal quarters (October 1, 2008, through December 31, 2010), and the temporary FMAP increase was extended by six months (January 1, 2011, through June 30, 2011) at a phased down level through P.L. 111-226. For more information about the temporary FMAP increase, see CRS Report RL32950, Medicaid's Federal Medical Assistance Percentage (FMAP), FY2013, by Alison Mitchell and Evelyne P. Baumrucker.

71 CRS calculations based on Form CMS-64 data from the Centers for Medicare & Medicaid.

72 CRS calculation based on Form CMS-64 data from the Centers for Medicare & Medicaid. The FY2011 CMS-64 data is not finalized, and the data used is as of April 16, 2012.

73 Does not add to 61% due to rounding.

74 Numbers may not exactly sum to totals, due to rounding. Anna Sommers, Arunabh Ghosh, and David Rousseau, Medicaid Enrollment and Spending by "Mandatory" and "Optional" Eligibility and Benefit Categories, Kaiser Commission on Medicaid and the Uninsured, June 2005.

75 Todd P. Gilmer and Richard G. Kronick, "Differences in the Volume of Services and in Prices Drive Big Variation in Medicaid Spending Among U.S. States and Regions," Health Affairs, vol. 30, no. 7 (July 2011).

76 Ibid.

77 To maximize the comparability of the sample across states, the study population was Medicaid-only disabled Medicaid enrollees on cash assistance that received Medicaid services on a fee-for-service basis. Todd P. Gilmer and Richard G. Kronick, "Differences in the Volume of Services and in Prices Drive Big Variation in Medicaid Spending Among U.S. States and Regions," Health Affairs, vol. 30, no. 7 (July 2011).

78 Historically, Medicaid eligibility was generally limited to low-income children, pregnant women, parents of dependent children, the elderly, and people with disabilities. For more information about the ACA changes to Medicaid, see CRS Report R41210, Medicaid and the State Children's Health Insurance Program (CHIP) Provisions in ACA: Summary and Timeline, by Evelyne P. Baumrucker et al.

79 Centers for Medicare & Medicaid Services, State Medicaid and CHIP Income Eligibility Standards Effective January 1, 2014, October 24, 2013.

80 States' decisions are based on CRS's monitoring of state activity through media outlets and state tracking of decisions done by CMS, State Refor(u)m, the Kaiser Family Foundation, the Advisory Board Company, and Avalere.

81 Figure reflects average annual enrollment. Congressional Budget Office, Updated Estimates for the Insurance Coverage Provisions of the Affordable Care Act, March 2012.

82 The difference in the estimated number of individuals covered by the ACA Medicaid expansion before and after the Supreme Court decision varies in each year between FY2014 to FY2022. The following is the difference between the two estimates in each year: FY2014

= 5 million, FY2015 = 3 million, FY2016 = 5 million, FY2017 = 4 million, FY2018 = 4 million, FY2019 = 4 million, FY2020 = 4 million, FY2021 = 4 million, and FY2022 = 4 million. (Congressional Budget Office, Updated Estimates for the Insurance Coverage Provisions of the Affordable Care Act, March 2012; Congressional Budget Office, The Budget and Economic Outlook: 2014 to 2024, February 2014.)

[83] Congressional Budget Office, The Budget and Economic Outlook: 2014 to 2024, February 2014.

[84] Ibid.

[85] For more information about the other ACA provisions impacting the Medicaid program, see CRS Report R41210, Medicaid and the State Children's Health Insurance Program (CHIP) Provisions in ACA: Summary and Timeline, by Evelyne P. Baumrucker et al.

[86] Community First Choice Option is a state plan option in which states can offer consumer-directed personal care attendant services and receive an increased federal match rate of 6 percentage points for doing so.

[87] The Money Follows the Person demonstration helps states rebalance their long-term care systems by transitioning people with Medicaid from institutions to the community.

[88] Congressional Budget Office, Selected CBO Publications Related to Health Care Legislation, 2009-2010, December 22, 2010.

[89] Office of Management and Budget, Historical Tables: Budget of the U.S. Government.

[90] National Commission on Fiscal Reform,The Moment of Truth: Report of the National Commission on Fiscal Responsibility and Reform, December 1, 2010.

[91] Debt Reduction Task Force, Restoring America's Future, November 2010.

[92] Department of Health and Human Services, Fiscal Year 2014 Budget in Brief: Strengthening Health and Opportunity for All Americans and Department of Health and Human Services' Centers for Medicare & Medicaid Services, Fiscal Year 2014 Justification of Estimates for Appropriations Committees.

[93] National Association of State Budget Officers, State Expenditure Report: Examining Fiscal 2011-2013 State Spending, 2013.

[94] The American Recovery and Reinvestment Act of 2009 (ARRA, P.L. 111-5) included a temporary increase to FMAP rates to help states maintain their Medicaid programs and free up funds that states would have otherwise used for Medicaid to address other state budgetary needs. The temporary FMAP rate increase was originally provided for nine fiscal quarters (October 1, 2008, through December 31, 2010), and the temporary FMAP rate increase was extended by six months (January 1, 2011, through June 30, 2011) at a phased down level through P.L. 111-226. For more information about the temporary FMAP rate increase, see CRS Report RL32950, Medicaid's Federal Medical Assistance Percentage (FMAP), FY2013, by Alison Mitchell and Evelyne P. Baumrucker.

[95] National Association of State Budget Officers, Fiscal Year 2010 State Expenditure Report: Examining Fiscal 2009- 2011 State Spending, December 2011; National Association of State Budget Officers, State Expenditure Report: Examining Fiscal 2011-2013 State Spending, 2013.

[96] U.S. Government Accountability Office, Medicaid: Improving Responsiveness to Federal Assistance to States During Economic Downturns, GAO-11-395, March 2011.

[97] Ibid.

[98] Lucy Dadayan and Donald Boyd, Strong Growth in the First Half; Softening Growth Outlook for the Rest of 2013, The Nelson A. Rockefeller Institute of Government at the University at Albany, State Revenue Report No. 93, December 2013.

[99] Kaiser Commission on Medicaid and the Uninsured, A Mid-Year State Medicaid Budget Update for FY 2012 and A Look Forward to FY2013, February 2012; Vernon K. Smith, Kathleen Gifford, Eileen Ellis, et al., Moving Ahead Amid Fiscal Challenges: A Look at Medicaid Spending, Coverage and Policy Trends, Results from a 50-State Medicaid Budget Survey for State Fiscal Years 2011 and 2012, Kaiser Commission on Medicaid and the Uninsured, October 2011; Vernon K. Smith, Robin Rudowitz, and Laura Snyder, Medicaid in a Historic Time of Transformation: Results from a 50-State Medicaid Budget Survey for State Fiscal Years 2013 and 2014, Kaiser Commission on Medicaid and the Uninsured, October 2013.

[100] For more information about the MOE requirements, see CRS Report R41835, Medicaid and CHIP Maintenance of Effort (MOE): Requirements and Responses, by Evelyne P. Baumrucker.

[101] Kaiser Commission on Medicaid and the Uninsured, A Mid-Year State Medicaid Budget Update for FY 2012 and A Look Forward to FY2013, February 2012; Vernon K. Smith, Kathleen Gifford, Eileen Ellis, et al., Moving Ahead Amid Fiscal Challenges: A Look at Medicaid Spending, Coverage and Policy Trends, Results from a 50-State Medicaid Budget Survey for State Fiscal Years 2011 and 2012, Kaiser Commission on Medicaid and the Uninsured, October 2011.

[102] Vernon K. Smith, Robin Rudowitz, and Laura Snyder, Medicaid in a Historic Time of Transformation: Results from a 50-State Medicaid Budget Survey for State Fiscal Years 2013 and 2014, Kaiser Commission on Medicaid and the Uninsured, October 2013.

[103] Kaiser Commission on Medicaid and the Uninsured, State Medicaid Agencies Prepare for Health Care Reform While Continuing to Face Challenges from the Recession. August 2010.

[104] Budget stabilization or "rainy day" funds allow states to set aside excess revenue for use in times of unexpected revenue shortfall or budget deficit. State Budget Crisis Task Force, Report of the State Budget Crisis Task Force, July 2012.

[105] U.S. Government Accountability Office, State and Local Governments' Fiscal Outlook: April 2012 Update, GAO12-523SP, April 2012. State Budget Crisis Task Force, Report of the State Budget Crisis Task Force, July 2012.

[106] Christopher J. Truffer, John D. Klemm, Christian J. Wolfe, et al., 2011 Actuarial Report on the Financial Outlook for Medicaid, Centers for Medicare & Medicaid Services' Office of the Actuary, March 2012.

[107] State Budget Crisis Task Force, Report of the State Budget Crisis Task Force, July 2012.

[108] While some states have expressed concerns about the fiscal challenge of funding the ACA Medicaid expansion, there are health and financial benefits associated with Medicaid coverage. A study of a Medicaid expansion in Oregon found that Medicaid coverage increased health care utilization (including both preventive care and hospitalizations), lower out-of-pocket medical expenditures and medical debt, and better self-reported physical and mental health. (Amy Finkelstein, Sarah Taubman, Bill Wright, et al., "The Oregon Health Insurance Experiment: Evidence from the First Year," National Bureau of Economic Research, July 2011.)

In: Medicaid Spending by States
Editor: Hank Milford

ISBN: 978-1-63463-538-7

Chapter 3

MEDICAID'S FEDERAL MEDICAL ASSISTANCE PERCENTAGE (FMAP), FY2014*

Alison Mitchell and Evelyne P. Baumrucker

SUMMARY

Medicaid is a means-tested entitlement program that finances the delivery of primary and acute medical services as well as long-term care. Medicaid is jointly funded by the federal government and the states. The federal government's share of a state's expenditures is called the federal medical assistance percentage (FMAP) rate. The remainder is referred to as the nonfederal share, or state share.

Generally determined annually, the FMAP formula is designed so that the federal government pays a larger portion of Medicaid costs in states with lower per capita incomes relative to the national average (and vice versa for states with higher per capita incomes). FMAP rates have a statutory minimum of 50% and a statutory maximum of 83%. For FY2014, regular FMAP rates range from 50.00% to 73.05%. The FMAP rate is used to reimburse states for the federal share of most Medicaid expenditures, but exceptions to the regular FMAP rate have been made for certain states, situations, populations, providers, and services.

* This is an edited, reformatted and augmented version of a Congressional Research Service publication R42941, prepared for Members and Committees of Congress, dated January 30, 2013.

Some recent issues related to FMAP include FMAP changes in the Patient Protection and Affordable Care Act (ACA, P.L. 111-148 as amended), federal deficit reduction proposals that would amend the FMAP rate, and the disaster-related FMAP adjustment.

The ACA contains a number of provisions affecting FMAP rates. Most notably, the ACA provides initial FMAP rates of up to 100% for certain "newly eligible" individuals. Also, under the ACA, "expansion states" receive an enhanced FMAP rate for certain individuals. In addition, ACA provides increased FMAP rates for certain disaster-affected states, primary care payment rate increases, specified preventive services and immunizations, smoking cessation services for pregnant women, specified home and community-based services, health home services for certain people with chronic conditions, home and community-based attendant services and supports, and state balancing incentive payments.

Since federal Medicaid expenditures are a large and growing portion of the federal budget, controlling federal Medicaid spending has been included in some federal deficit reduction proposals. Some of the federal deficit reduction proposals include provisions that would amend the current FMAP structure through either a blended FMAP or a reduction to the statutory FMAP floor.

The ACA included a provision providing a disaster-recovery FMAP adjustment for states that have experienced a major, statewide disaster. Louisiana is the only state that has been eligible for the disaster-recovery adjusted FMAP since the fourth quarter of FY2011 (when the adjustment was first available). Both the Middle Class Tax Relief and Job Creation Act of 2012 (P.L. 112-96) and the Moving Ahead for Progress in the 21st Century Act (MAP-21, P.L. 112-141) amended the formula for the disaster-recovery adjusted FMAP.

This report describes the FMAP calculation used to reimburse states for most Medicaid expenditures, and it lists the statutory exceptions to the regular FMAP rate. In addition, this report discusses other FMAP-related issues, including FMAP changes in ACA, federal deficit reduction proposals affecting the FMAP rate, and the disaster-recovery FMAP adjustment.

INTRODUCTION

Medicaid is a means-tested entitlement program that finances the delivery of primary and acute medical services as well as long-term care.[1] Medicaid is jointly funded by the federal government and the states. Participation in Medicaid is voluntary for states, though all states, the District of Columbia, and the territories choose to participate. Each state designs and administers its own version of Medicaid under broad federal rules. While states that choose to participate in Medicaid must comply with all federal mandated requirements, state variability is the rule rather than the exception in terms of eligibility levels, covered services, and how those services are reimbursed and delivered. Historically, eligibility was generally limited to low-income children, pregnant women, parents of dependent children, the elderly, and people with disabilities; however, recent changes will soon add coverage for individuals under the age of 65 with income up to 133% of the federal poverty level.[2] The federal government pays a share of each state's Medicaid costs; states must contribute the remaining portion in order to qualify for federal funds.[3]

This report describes the federal medical assistance percentage (FMAP) calculation used to reimburse states for most Medicaid expenditures, and it lists the statutory exceptions to the regular FMAP rate. In addition, this report discusses other FMAP-related issues, including FMAP changes in the Patient Protection and Affordable Care Act (ACA, P.L. 111-148 as amended), federal deficit reduction proposals that would amend the FMAP rate, and the disaster-recovery FMAP adjustment.

THE FEDERAL MEDICAL ASSISTANCE PERCENTAGE

The federal government's share of most Medicaid service costs is determined by the FMAP rate, which varies by state and is determined by a formula set in statute. The FMAP rate is used to reimburse states for the federal share of most Medicaid expenditures, but exceptions to the regular FMAP rate have been made for certain states, situations, populations, providers, and services.[4]

An enhanced FMAP (E-FMAP) rate is provided for both services and administration under the State Children's Health Insurance Program (CHIP), subject to the availability of funds from a state's federal allotment for CHIP. When a state expands its Medicaid program using CHIP funds (rather than Medicaid funds), the E-FMAP rate applies and is paid out of the state's federal allotment. The E-FMAP rate is calculated by reducing the state share under the regular FMAP rate by 30%.[5]

The FMAP rate is also used in determining the phased-down state contribution ("clawback") for Medicare Part D, the federal share of certain child support enforcement collections, Temporary Assistance for Needy Families (TANF) contingency funds, a portion of the Child Care and

Development Fund (CCDF), and foster care and adoption assistance under Title IV-E of the Social Security Act.

How FMAP Rates Are Calculated

The FMAP formula compares each state's per capita income relative to U.S. per capita income. The formula provides higher reimbursement to states with lower incomes (with a statutory maximum of 83%) and lower reimbursement to states with higher incomes (with a statutory minimum of 50%). The formula[6] for a given state is:

$$FMAP_{state} = 1 - ((\text{Per capita income}_{state})^2/(\text{Per capita income}_{U.S.})^2 * 0.45)$$

The use of the 0.45 factor in the formula is designed to ensure that a state with per capita income equal to the U.S. average receives an FMAP rate of 55% (i.e., state share of 45%). In addition, the formula's squaring of income provides higher FMAP rates to states with below-average incomes (and vice versa, subject to the 50% minimum).[7]

The Department of Health & Human Services (HHS) usually publishes FMAP rates for an upcoming fiscal year in the *Federal Register* during the preceding November. This time lag between announcement and implementation provides an opportunity for states to adjust to FMAP rate changes, but it also means that the per capita income amounts used to calculate FMAP rates for a given fiscal year are several years old by the time the FMAP rates take effect.

In the *Appendix* to this report, *Table A-1* shows regular FMAP rates for each of the 50 states and the District of Columbia from FY2006-FY2014.

Data Used to Calculate State FMAP Rates

As specified in Section 1905(b) of the Social Security Act, the per capita income amounts used in the FMAP formula are equal to the average of the three most recent calendar years of data available from the Department of Commerce. In its FY2014 FMAP calculations, HHS used state per capita personal income data for 2009, 2010, and 2011 that became available from the Department of Commerce's Bureau of Economic Analysis (BEA) in

September 2012. The use of a three-year average helps to moderate fluctuations in a state's FMAP rate over time.

BEA revises its most recent estimates of state per capita personal income on an annual basis to incorporate revised and newly available source data on population and income.[8] It also undertakes a comprehensive data revision—reflecting methodological and other changes—every few years that may result in upward and downward revisions to each of the component parts of personal income (as defined in BEA's national income and product accounts, or NIPA). These components include:

- earnings (wages and salaries, employer contributions for employee pension and insurance funds, and proprietors' income);
- dividends, interest, and rent; and
- personal current transfer receipts (e.g., government social benefits such as Social Security, Medicare, Medicaid, state unemployment insurance).[9]

As a result of these annual and comprehensive revisions, it is often the case that the value of a state's per capita personal income for a given year will change over time. For example, the 2009 state per capita personal income data published by BEA in September 2011 (used in the calculation of FY2013 FMAP rates) differed from the 2009 state per capita personal income data published in September 2012 (used in the calculation of FY2014 FMAP rates).

It should be noted that the NIPA definition of personal income used by BEA is not the same as the definition used for personal income tax purposes. Among other differences, NIPA personal income excludes capital gains (or losses) and includes transfer receipts (e.g., government social benefits), while income for tax purposes includes capital gains (or losses) and excludes most of these transfers.

Factors that Affect FMAP Rates

Several factors affect states' FMAP rates. The first is the nature of the state economy and, to the extent possible, a state's ability to respond to economic changes (i.e., downturns or upturns). The impact on a particular state of a national economic downturn or upturn will be related to the structure of the state economy and its business sectors. For example, a national decline in automobile sales, while having an impact on all state economies, will have a larger impact in states that manufacture automobiles as production is reduced and workers are laid off.

Second, the FMAP formula relies on per capita personal income *in relation to the U.S. average per capita personal income.* The national economy is basically the sum of all state economies. As a result, the national response to an economic change is the sum of the state responses to economic change. If more states (or larger states) experience an economic decline, the national economy reflects this decline to some extent. However, the national decline will be lower than some states' declines because the total decline has been offset by states with small decreases or even increases (i.e., states with growing economies). The U.S. per capita personal income, because of this balancing of positive and negative, has only a small percentage change each year. Since the FMAP formula compares state changes in per capita personal income (which can have large changes each year) to the U.S. per capita personal income, this comparison can result in significant state FMAP rate changes.

In addition to annual revisions of per capita personal income data, comprehensive NIPA revisions undertaken every four to five years may also influence regular FMAP rates (e.g., because of changes in the definition of personal income). The impact on FMAP rates will depend on whether the changes are broad (affecting all states) or more selective (affecting only certain states or industries).

FY2014 Regular FMAP Rates

Regular FMAP rates for FY2014 (the federal fiscal year that begins on October 1, 2013) were calculated and published November 30, 2012, in the *Federal Register.*[10] In the *Appendix* to this report, *Table A-1* shows regular FMAP rates for each of the 50 states and the District of Columbia for FY2006 through FY2014. *Figure 1* shows the state distribution of regular FMAP rates for FY2014. Fifteen states will have the statutory minimum FMAP rate of 50.00% (Rhode Island is very close at 50.11%), and Mississippi will have the highest FMAP rate of 73.05%.

As shown in *Figure 1*, from FY2013 to FY2014, the regular FMAP rates for 36 states will change, while the regular FMAP rates for the remaining 15 states (including the District of Columbia) will remain the same.[11]

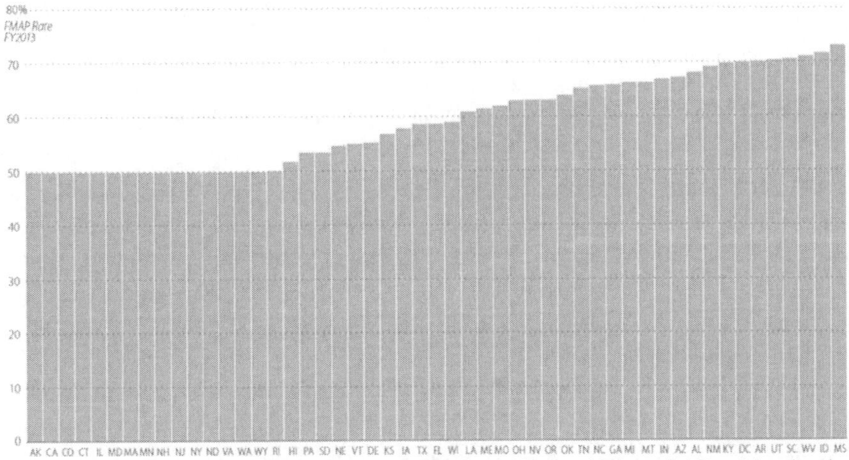

Source: Department of Health and Human Services, "Federal Financial Participation in State Assistance Expenditures; Federal Matching Shares for Medicaid, the Children's Health Insurance Program, and Aid to Needy Aged, Blind, or Disabled Persons for October 1, 2013 Through September 30, 2014," 77 Federal Register 71420, November 30, 2012.

Note: State-by-state FY2014 regular FMAP rates are listed in Table A-1.

Figure 1. State Distribution of Regular FMAP Rates. FY2014

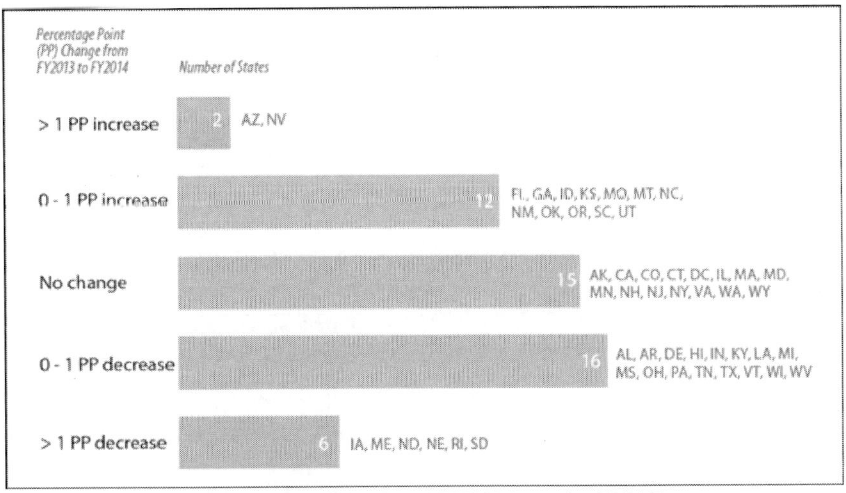

Source: Prepared by CRS using FY2013 and FY2014 regular FMAP rates.

Note: Specific FMAP rate changes for each state are listed in Table A-1.

Figure 2. FMAP Rate Changes for States from FY2013 to FY2014.

For most of the states experiencing an FMAP rate change from FY2013 to FY2014, the change will be less than one percentage point. The regular FMAP rate for 12 states will increase by as much as one percentage point, and the FMAP rate for 16 states will decrease by as much as one percentage point.

For states that will experience an FMAP rate change greater than one percentage point from FY2013 to FY2014, two states will experience an FMAP rate increase of greater than one percentage point, and six states will experience an FMAP rate decrease of greater than one percentage point. Nevada will have the largest FMAP rate increase with a 3.36 percentage point increase, and South Dakota will have the largest FMAP rate decrease with a 2.65 percentage point decrease.

Two states will have FY2014 FMAP rates that are not calculated according to the regular FMAP formula: the District of Columbia and Louisiana. The FMAP rate for the District of Columbia has been set in statute at 70% since 1998, and Louisiana will receive a disaster-recovery FMAP adjustment (discussed in further detail below) increase over its FY2014 regular FMAP rate.

FMAP Exceptions

Although FMAP rates are generally determined by the formula described above, *Table 1* lists exceptions that have been added to the Medicaid statute over the years. *Table 1* identifies whether the exception is a current (i.e., the exception currently applies), future (i.e., the exception will apply beginning at the specified date), or past (i.e., the exception no longer applies) FMAP rate exception.

Table 1. Exceptions to the Regular FMAP Rates for Medicaid

Exception	Description	Citations	Past, Current, or Future Exception
Territories and Certain States			
Territories	As of July 1, 2011, FMAP rates for the territories (Puerto Rico, American Samoa, the Northern Mariana Islands, Guam, and the Virgin Islands) were increased from	Most recently P.L. 111-148, as amended by P.L. 111-152; SSA §1905(b), 1108(f)	Current

Exception	Description	Citations	Past, Current, or Future Exception
	50% to 55%. Unlike the 50 states and the District of Columbia, the territories are subject to federal spending caps. The 55% also applies for purposes of computing the enhanced FMAP rate for CHIP.	and (g)	
District of Columbia	As of FY1998, the District of Columbia's FMAP rate is set at 70% (without this exception, it would be at the statutory minimum of 50%). The 70% also applies for purposes of computing the enhanced FMAP rate for CHIP.	P.L. 105-33; SSA §1905(b)	Current
Alaska	Alaska's FMAP rate was set in statute for FY1998-FY2000 at 59.80%; used an alternative formula for FY2001-FY2005 that reduced the state's per capita income by 5% (thereby increasing its FMAP rate); and was held at its FY2005 level for FY2006-FY2007. These provisions also applied for purposes of computing the enhanced FMAP rate for CHIP.	P.L. 105-33 §4725(a); P.L. 106-554 Appendix F §706; P.L. 109-171 §6053(a)	Past
Special Situations			
Adjustment for disaster recovery	Beginning in CY2011, a disaster-recovery FMAP adjustment is available for states in which (1) during one of the preceding seven years, the President declared a major disaster under the Stafford Act and every county in the state warranted at least public assistance under that act and (2) the regular FMAP rate declines by a specified amount. To trigger the adjustment, a state's regular FMAP rate must be at least three percentage points less than such state's last year's regular FMAP rate plus (if applicable) any hold harmless increase under P.L.	P.L. 111-148, as amended by P.L. 111-152, P.L. 112-96 P.L, and 112-141; SSA §1905(aa); 75 *Federal Register* 80501 (December 22, 2010)	Current

Table 1. (Continued)

Exception	Description	Citations	Past, Current, or Future Exception
	111-5; the adjustment is an FMAP rate increase equal to 50% of the difference between the two. To continue receiving the adjustment, the state's regular FMAP rate must be at least three percentage points less than last year's adjusted FMAP rate; the adjustment is an FMAP rate increase equal to 25% of the difference between the two. (Discussed in further detail in the text.)		
Adjustment for certain employer contributions	As of FY2006, significantly disproportionate employer pension and insurance fund contributions will be excluded from the calculation of Medicaid FMAP rates. This will have the effect of reducing certain states' per capita personal income relative to the national average, which in turn could increase their Medicaid FMAP rates. Any identifiable employer contributions towards pensions or other employee insurance funds are considered to be significantly disproportionate if the increase in the amount of employer contributions accrued to residents of a state exceeds 25% of the total increase in personal income in that state for the year involved. To date, no state has qualified for this adjustment.	P.L. 111-3 §614; 75 *Federal Register* 63482 (October 15, 2010)	Current
State fiscal relief, FY2009-FY2011	FMAP rates were increased from the first quarter of FY2009 through the third quarter of FY2011, providing states with more than $100 billion (about $84 billion for	P.L. 111-5 §5001, as amended by P.L. 111-226 §201	Past

Exception	Description	Citations	Past, Current, or Future Exception
	the original provision and $16 billion for a six-month extension) in additional funds. All states received a hold harmless to prevent any decline in regular FMAP rates and an across-the-board increase of 6.2 percentage points until the last two quarters of the period, at which point the across-the-board percentage point increase phased down to 3.2 and then 1.2; qualifying states received an additional unemployment-related increase. Each territory could choose between an FMAP increase of 6.2 percentage points along with a 15% increase in its spending cap, or its regular FMAP rate along with a 30% increase in its cap; all chose the latter. States were required to meet certain requirements in order to receive the increase.		
Adjustment for Hurricane Katrina	In computing FMAP rates for any year after 2006 for a state that the Secretary of HHS determines has a significant number of Hurricane Katrina evacuees as of October 1, 2005, the Secretary must disregard such evacuees and their incomes. Although it was labeled as a "hold harmless for Katrina impact," the provision language required evacuees to be disregarded even if their inclusion would increase a state's FMAP rate. Due to lags in the availability of data used to calculate FMAP rates, FY2008 was the first year to which the provision applied. HHS proposed and finalized a methodology that.	P.L. 109-171 §6053(b); 72 *Federal Register* 3391 (January 25, 2007) and 44146 (August 7, 2007)	Past

Table 1. (Continued)

Exception	Description	Citations	Past, Current, or Future Exception
	prevented the lowering of any FY2008 FMAP rates and increased the FY2008 FMAP rate for one state (Texas). The methodology took advantage of a data timing issue that does not apply after FY2008. HHS had initially expressed concern that some states could see lower FMAP rates in later years as a result of the provision, but the final methodology indicated that there is no reliable way to track the number and income of evacuees on an ongoing basis and therefore no basis for adjusting FMAP rates after FY2008. The provision also applied for purposes of computing the enhanced FMAP rate for CHIP		
State fiscal relief, FY2003-FY2004	FMAP rates for the last two quarters of FY2003 and the first three quarters of FY2004 were not allowed to decline (i.e., were held harmless) and were increased by an additional 2.95 percentage points, providing states with about $10 billion in additional funds (they also received $10 billion in direct grants). Although Medicaid disproportionate share hospital (DSH) payments are reimbursed using the FMAP rate, the increase did not apply to DSH. States had to meet certain requirements in order to receive an increase (e.g., they could not restrict eligibility after a specified date).	P.L. 108-27 §401(a)	Past
Certain Populations			
"Newly eligible" individuals	Historically, Medicaid eligibility generally has been limited to low-	P.L. 111-148, as amended by P.L.	Future

Exception	Description	Citations	Past, Current, or Future Exception
enrolled in new eligibility group through 133% FPL	income individuals who fall into specified categories (typically children, parents, pregnant women, disabled, and elderly). As of CY2014, Medicaid coverage will be available to individuals under a new eligibility group for nonelderly, nonpregnant adults at or below 133% FPL at state option. The law specifies an income disregard in the amount of 5% FPL will be deducted from an individual's income when determining Medicaid eligibility based on MAGI, thus the effective upper income eligibility threshold for such individuals in this new eligibility group will be 138% FPL. An increased FMAP rate will be provided for services rendered to "newly eligible" individuals in this group. The "newly eligible" are defined as those who would not have been eligible for Medicaid in the state as of 12/1/2009 or were eligible under a waiver but not enrolled because of limits or caps on waiver enrollment. The FMAP rates for "newly eligible" individuals will equal: CY2014-CY2016 = 100%; CY2017 = 95%; CY2018 = 94%; CY2019 = 93%; CY2020+ = 90%.	111-152; SSA §1905(y)	
"Expansion state" individuals enrolled in new eligibility group through 133% FPL	Although Medicaid eligibility has generally been limited to certain categories of individuals, some states provide health coverage for all low-income individuals using Medicaid waivers. As a result, they have few or no individuals who will qualify for the	P.L. 111-148, as amended by P.L. 111-152; SSA §1905(z)(2)	Future

Table 1. (Continued)

Exception	Description	Citations	Past, Current, or Future Exception
	"newly eligible" FMAP rate beginning in CY2014. To address this issue, as of CY2014, an increased FMAP rate will be provided for individuals in "expansion states" who were eligible for Medicaid as of 3/23/10 (P.L. 111-148's enactment date) in the new eligibility group for nonelderly, nonpregnant adults at or below 133% FPL. "Expansion states" are defined as those that, as of 3/23/2010, offered health benefits coverage meeting certain criteria statewide to parents and nonpregnant childless adults at least through 100% FPL. The formula used to calculate "expansion state" FMAP rates is [regular FMAP + (newly eligible FMAP – regular FMAP) * transition percentage equal to 50% in CY2014, 60% in CY2015, 70% in CY2016, 80% in CY2017, 90% in CY2018, and 100% in CY2019+] will lead the "expansion state" FMAP rates to vary based on a state's regular FMAP rate until CY2019, at which point they will equal "newly eligible" FMAP rates: CY2014 = at least 75%; CY2015 = at least 80%; CY2016 = at least 85%; CY2017 = at least 86%; CY2018 = at least 90%; CY2019 = 93%; CY2020+ = 90%.		
Other "expansion state" individuals	During CY2014 and CY2015, an FMAP rate increase of 2.2 percentage points is available for "expansion states" that (1) the	P.L. 111-148, as amended by P.L. 111-152; SSA §1905(z)(1)	Future

Exception	Description	Citations	Past, Current, or Future Exception
	Secretary of HHS determines will not receive any FMAP rate increase for "newly eligible" individuals and (2) have not been approved to divert Medicaid disproportionate share hospital funds to pay for the cost of health coverage under a waiver in effect as of July 2009. The FMAP rate increase applies to those who are *not* "newly eligible" individuals as described in relation to the new eligibility group for nonelderly, nonpregnant adults at or below 133% FPL. It appears that Vermont meets the criteria for this increase.		
Certain women with breast or cervical cancer	For states that opt to cover certain women with breast or cervical cancer who do not qualify for Medicaid under a mandatory eligibility pathway and are otherwise uninsured, expenditures for these women are reimbursed using the enhanced FMAP rate that applies to CHIP.	P.L. 106-354, as amended by P.L. 107-121; SSA §1905(b)	Current
Qualifying Individuals program	States are required to pay Medicare Part B premiums for Medicare beneficiaries with income between 120% and 135% FPL and limited assets (referred to as "qualifying individuals"), up to a specified dollar allotment. They receive 100% federal reimbursement for these costs, which are financed at the federal level by a transfer of funds from Medicare to Medicaid. This provision has been extended numerous times and is currently funded through December 31, 2013.	P.L. 105-33, most recently extended via P.L. 112-240; SSA §1933(d)	Current

Table 1. (Continued)

Exception	Description	Citations	Past, Current, or Future Exception
Certain Providers			
Primary care payment rates	During CY2013 and CY2014, states are required to provide Medicaid payments that are at or above Medicare rates for primary care services (defined as evaluation and management and certain administration of immunizations) furnished by a physician with a primary specialty designation of family, general internal, or pediatric medicine. States will receive 100% federal reimbursement for expenditures attributable to the amount by which Medicare exceeds their Medicaid payment rates in effect on 7/1/2009.	P.L. 111-148, as amended by P.L. 111-152; SSA §1902(a)(13)(C); 77 *Federal Register* 66670.	Current
Indian Health Service facility	States receive 100% federal reimbursement for services provided through an Indian Health Service facility.	P.L. 94-437; SSA §1905(b)	Current
Certain Services			
Certain preventive services and immunizations	As of CY2013, states that opt to cover—with no cost sharing—clinical preventive services recommended with a grade of A or B by the United States Preventive Services Task Force (USPSTF) and adult immunizations recommended by the Advisory Committee on Immunization Practices (ACIP) will receive a one percentage point increase in their FMAP rate for those services.	P.L. 111-148, as amended by P.L. 111-152; SSA §1905(b)	Current
Smoking cessation for pregnant women	As of CY2013, states that opt to cover USPSTF preventive services and ACIP adult immunizations as noted above will also receive a one percentage point increase in their	P.L. 111-148, as amended by P.L. 111-152; SSA §1905(b)	Current

Exception	Description	Citations	Past, Current, or Future Exception
	FMAP rate for smoking cessation services that are mandatory for pregnant women.		
Family planning	States receive 90% federal reimbursement for family planning services and supplies.	P.L. 92-603; SSA §1903(a)(5)	Current
Health homes	As of CY2011, states have a new option for providing "health home" and associated services to certain individuals with chronic conditions. They will receive 90% federal reimbursement for these services for the first eight quarters that the health home option is in effect in the state.	P.L. 111-148, as amended by P.L. 111-152; SSA §1945(c)(1)	Current
Home and communitybased attendant services and supports	As of FY2011, states have a new option for providing home and community-based attendant services and supports for certain individuals at or below 150% FPL, or a higher income level applicable to those who require an institutional level of care. They will receive a six percentage point increase in their regular FMAP rate for these services.	P.L. 111-148, as amended by P.L. 111-152; SSA §1915(k)(2)	Current
State balancing incentive payments	During FY2011 FY2015, state balancing incentive payments are available under certain conditions for states in which less than 50% of Medicaid expenditures for long-term services and supports (LTSS) are non-institutional. Qualifying states with less than 25% non-institutional LTSS must plan to achieve a 25% target and can receive a five percentage point increase in their FMAP rate for non-institutional LTSS; those with less than 50% must plan to achieve a 50% target and can receive a two	P.L. 111-148, as amended by P.L. 111-152, §10202	Current

Table 1. (Continued)

Exception	Description	Citations	Past, Current, or Future Exception
	percentage point increase. Federal spending on these increased FMAP rates is limited to $3 billion during the period.		
Administrative Activities			
Training of Medical Personnel	States receive a 75% FMAP rate for costs attributable to compensation or training of skilled professional medical personnel, and staff directly supporting such personnel.	SSA §1903(a)(2)(A)&(B)	Current
Immigration Verification System	States receive 100% federal reimbursement for the cost of implementation and operation of an immigration status verification system.	SSA §1903(a)(4)	Current
Fraud Control Unit	States receive 75% FMAP rate for state expenditures related to the operation of a state Medicaid fraud control unit.	SSA §1903(a)(6)	Current
Preadmission Screening	State expenditures attributable to preadmission screening and resident review for individuals with mental illness or mental retardation who are admitted to a nursing facility receive 75% FMAP rate.	SSA §1903(a)(2)(C)	Current
Survey and Certification	States receive 75% FMAP rate for state expenditures related to survey and certification of nursing facilities.	SSA §1903(a)(2)(D)	Current
Managed Care Review Activities	States receive 75% FMAP rate for state expenditures related to performance of medical and utilization review activities or external independent review of managed care activities.	SSA §1903(a)(3)(C)	Current
Claims and Eligibility	States receive 90% FMAP rate for the design, development, or	SSA §1903(a)(3)(A) and (B); 76 *Federal*	Current

Exception	Description	Citations	Past, Current, or Future Exception
Systems	installation of mechanized claims systems and 75% FMAP rate for operating mechanized claims systems. Both federal reimbursement percentages are subject to certain criteria set by the Secretary of HHS, which includes whether the activity is likely to provide more efficient, economical, and effective administration of claims processing. CMS published a final rule to amend the definition of Mechanized Claims Processing and Information Retrieval systems to include systems used for eligibility determination, enrollment, and eligibility reporting activities thereby making the 90% FMAP rate available for the design, development and installation or enhancement of eligibility determination systems until December 31, 2015, and 75% FMAP rate for maintenance and operations available for such systems beyond that date as long as certain requirements are met.	*Register* 21950 (April 19, 2011)	
Translation or Interpretation Services	Administrative expenditures for translation or interpretation services in connection with the "enrollment of, retention of, and use of services" under Medicaid receive 75% FMAP rate. For CHIP, the increased match is 75%, or the state's enhanced FMAP rate plus 5 percentage points, whichever is higher, and the CHIP increased match is subject to the 10% cap on administrative expenditures. The increased FMAP rate for translation or interpretation	P.L. 111-3; SSA §1903(a)(2)(E); State Medicaid Director Letter, State Health Official 10-007, CHIPRA 18, July 1, 2010.	Current

Table 1. (Continued)

Exception	Description	Citations	Past, Current, or Future Exception
	services is only available for eligible expenditures claimed as administrative and not expenditures claimed as medical assistance-related (which receive each state's regular FMAP rate).		
General Administration	Remaining state expenditures found necessary for the proper and efficient administration of the state plan receive a 50% FMAP rate.	SSA §1903(a)(7)	Current

Source: Congressional Research Service, based on sources noted in the table.

Notes: Unless noted, exceptions do not apply for purposes of computing the enhanced FMAP rate for CHIP. SSA = Social Security Act; FPL = federal poverty level; CHIPRA = Children's Health Insurance Program Reauthorization Act.

Recent Issues

Some recent issues related to the FMAP rate include FMAP changes in the ACA, federal deficit reduction proposals impacting the FMAP rate, and the disaster-related FMAP adjustment.

FMAP Changes in the ACA

The Medicaid provisions in ACA represent the most considerable reform to Medicaid since its enactment in 1965. The most noteworthy change begins in 2014, or sooner at state option, when the ACA expands Medicaid to include a new mandatory eligibility group: all adults under age 65 with income up to 133% of the federal poverty level (FPL) (effectively 138% FPL with the Modified Adjusted Gross Income or MAGI 5% FPL income disregard).[12] Originally, it was assumed that all states would implement the ACA Medicaid expansion in 2014 as required by statute because implementing the ACA Medicaid expansion was required in order for states to receive any federal Medicaid funding. However, on June 28, 2012, the United States Supreme

Court issued its decision in *National Federation of Independent Business (NFIB) v. Sebelius*[13] finding that the federal government cannot terminate the federal Medicaid funding a state receives for its current Medicaid program if a state refuses to implement the ACA Medicaid expansion. If a state accepts the new ACA Medicaid expansion funds, it must abide by the new expansion coverage rules. However, based on the Court's opinion, it appears that a state can refuse to participate in the ACA Medicaid expansion without losing any of its current federal Medicaid matching funds.[14]

While not all states are expected to implement the ACA Medicaid expansion, the Congressional Budget Office (CBO) estimates the Medicaid expansion will increase Medicaid enrollment by 7 million in FY2014, which is a 20% increase over the Medicaid enrollment estimated for FY2014 without the ACA Medicaid expansion.[15] As a result, the expansion will significantly increase Medicaid expenditures, and the federal government will cover a vast majority of the costs for individuals who are "newly eligible" due to ACA.

ACA contains a number of provisions that affect FMAP rates, such as the "newly eligible" FMAP rates, the "expansion state" FMAP rates, and other FMAP rate changes discussed below.

"Newly Eligible" FMAP Rates. An increased FMAP rate will be provided for "newly eligible" individuals who will gain Medicaid eligibility due to the ACA Medicaid expansion. The "newly eligible" are defined as nonelderly, nonpregnant adults with family income below 133% FPL who would not have been eligible for Medicaid in the state as of December 1, 2009, or were eligible under a waiver but not enrolled because of limits or caps on waiver enrollment. States will receive 100% FMAP rate for the cost of providing benchmark or benchmark-equivalent coverage[16] to "newly eligible" individuals, from 2014 through 2016. For "newly eligible" individuals, the FMAP rate will phase down to 95% in 2017, 94% in 2018, 93% in 2019, and 90% afterward (See *Table 2).*[17]

"Expansion State" FMAP Rates. Although Medicaid eligibility has generally been limited to certain categories of individuals, some states provide health coverage for all low-income individuals using Medicaid waivers. As a result, they have few or no individuals who will qualify for the "newly eligible" FMAP rate. As of CY2014, these states will receive an increased FMAP rate, which is referred to as the "expansion states" FMAP rate.

"Expansion states" are defined as those that, as of March 23, 2010 (ACA's enactment date), provided health benefits coverage meeting certain criteria[18] statewide to parents and nonpregnant childless adults at least through 100% FPL. Although HHS will make the official determination, one source suggests that 11 states (Arizona, Delaware, Hawaii, Maine, Massachusetts, Minnesota, New York, Pennsylvania, Vermont, Washington, and Wisconsin) and the District of Columbia might meet the definition of an "expansion state."[19]

Table 2. FMAP Rates for ACA Medicaid Expansion

	2014	2015	2016	2017	2018	2019	2020+
"Newly eligible" Adults in all States	100%	100%	100%	95%	94%	93%	90%
Certain Individuals in "Expansion states"	75%-92%	80%-93%	85%-95%	86%-93%	90%-93%	93%	90%

Source: Prepared by CRS.

Note: For the calculation of the "expansion state" FMAP rates, the lower bound is a state with a regular FMAP rate of 50% (which is the statutory minimum), and the upper bound is a state with a regular FMAP rate of 83% (which is the statutory maximum).

The "expansion state" FMAP rate will be available for individuals in "expansion states" who were eligible for Medicaid on March 23, 2010 and are in the new eligibility group for nonelderly, nonpregnant adults at or below 133% FPL. The formula[20] used to calculate the "expansion state" FMAP rates is based on a state's regular FMAP rate, so the "expansion state" FMAP rates will vary from state to state until CY2019, at which point the "newly eligible" FMAP rates and the "expansion state" FMAP rates will both be equal (see *Table 2*).

"Expansion states" are not excluded from receiving the "newly eligible" FMAP rates. Populations in an "expansion state" that meet the definition for the "newly eligible" FMAP rate will receive the "newly eligible" FMAP rate. For example, an "expansion state" that currently provides Medicaid coverage to childless adults and parents up to 100% FPL that chooses to implement the ACA Medicaid expansion will receive the higher "newly eligible" FMAP rate for individuals between 100% and 133% FPL. Also, "expansion states" will receive the "newly eligible" FMAP rate for individuals who received limited Medicaid benefits. In addition, "expansion states" that provided state-funded health benefits coverage will receive the "newly eligible" FMAP rate for individuals previously covered by the state-only program.[21]

Additional FMAP Increase for Certain "Expansion States." During CY2014 and CY2015, an FMAP rate increase of 2.2 percentage points is available for "expansion states" that (1) the Secretary of HHS determines will not receive any FMAP rate increase for "newly eligible" individuals and (2) have not been approved to divert Medicaid disproportionate share hospital funds to pay for the cost of health coverage under a waiver in effect as of July 2009. The FMAP rate increase applies to those who are *not* "newly eligible" individuals as described in relation to the new eligibility group for nonelderly, nonpregnant adults at or below 133% FPL. It appears that Vermont meets the criteria for this increase.

Additional Medicaid Changes. As noted in *Table 1*, ACA also provides—subject to various requirements—an increased FMAP rate for certain disaster-affected states, primary care payment rate increases, specified preventive services and immunizations, smoking cessation services for pregnant women, specified home and community-based services, health home services for certain people with chronic conditions, home and community-based attendant services and supports, and state balancing incentive payments. Three of these FMAP provisions went into effect on January 1, 2013: primary care payment rate increases, specified preventive services and immunizations, smoking cessation services for pregnant women. The other provisions have been in place for the past few years.

CHIP. Prior to ACA, federal CHIP allotments were provided through FY2013 and states received reimbursement for CHIP expenditures based on the E-FMAP rate described at the beginning of this report. Under ACA, the E FMAP rate for CHIP expenditures in FY2016-FY2019 will be increased by 23 percentage points, up to 100%.[22] ACA also provides new federal CHIP allotments for FY2014 and FY2015. However, no federal CHIP allotments are provided during the period in which the 23 percentage point increase in the E-FMAP rate is slated to be in effect.

Federal Deficit Reduction

In a typical year, the federal government funds roughly 57% of the total cost for Medicaid,[23] and federal Medicaid expenditures account for almost 8% of all federal spending.[24] In FY2013, federal Medicaid payments to states are estimated to amount to $276 billion.[25] Federal Medicaid payments are anticipated to grow significantly beginning in FY2014 due to the expansion of Medicaid eligibility provided in the ACA.[26] As a percentage of gross domestic product (GDP), federal Medicaid expenditures are expected to increase from about 1.7% of GDP in FY2013 to 2.4% of GDP in FY2022.[27] As a result, controlling federal Medicaid spending has been a focus of federal deficit reduction proposals, and amending the FMAP structure has been identified as a way to reduce federal Medicaid spending by a reduction to the statutory FMAP floor.

Reduce the FMAP Floor

As mentioned above, the FMAP has a statutory maximum of 83% and a statutory minimum of 50%. In its *Choices for Deficit Reduction* report, CBO provided estimates for a series of options that Congress may choose to examine as it considers deficit reduction. One such option would reduce federal Medicaid spending by reducing the statutory FMAP floor, and CBO estimates this option would save $20 billion in federal Medicaid expenditures in FY2020.[28]

Regular FMAP rates for FY2014 range from 50% (15 states) to 73% (Mississippi). If this option were in place for FY2014, it would impact the 15 states that have FMAP rates of 50%. The other 35 states and the District of Columbia would not be impacted by this option.

Disaster-Recovery Adjusted FMAP Rate

The ACA added a disaster-recovery FMAP adjustment for states that have experienced a major, statewide disaster. This adjustment was available to states beginning the fourth quarter of FY2011.[29]

There are two criteria for states to qualify for the disaster-recovery FMAP adjustment. First, during the preceding seven years, the President must have declared a major disaster under the Stafford Act in the state where every county in the state was eligible for public assistance from the federal government. Second, the state's regular FMAP rate must have declined at least three percentage points from the prior year's FMAP rate.[30]

In the first year a state qualifies for the disaster-recovery adjusted FMAP rate, the FMAP rate shall be equal to the regular FMAP rate as determined for the fiscal year, plus 50% of the difference between the current year's regular FMAP rate and the preceding year's FMAP rate. For the second and subsequent years a state qualifies for the adjustment, the FMAP rate shall be equal to the state's regular FMAP rate for that year plus 25% of the difference between the current year's regular FMAP rate and the preceding year's disaster-recovery adjusted FMAP rate.

Originally (i.e., as enacted by the ACA), for the second and subsequent years, the FMAP increase was applied to the prior year's disaster-recovery adjusted FMAP. However, this caused the state's FMAP rate to increase, rather than phase down as intended, each year a state qualifies for the adjustment. As a result, Section 3204 of the Middle Class Tax Relief and Job Creation Act of 2012 (P.L. 112-96) revised the formula so that for the second and subsequent years the increase will be applied to the regular FMAP as determined for the fiscal year. This provision had an effective date of October 1, 2013. The effective date was later amended by Section 100123 of the Moving Ahead for Progress in the 21st Century Act (MAP-21, P.L. 112-141) to October 1, 2012. In addition, MAP-21 amended the formula for FY2013 by changing the adjustment factor from 25% to 50% for only FY2013.

Louisiana was the only state that met both requirements for FY2011, FY2012, FY2013, and FY2014. *Table 3* shows the calculation for Louisiana's disaster-recovery adjusted FMAP rate for each of those years.

Table 3. Calculation for Louisiana's Disaster-Recovery Adjusted FMAP Rate

First Year of Disaster-Recovery Adjustment					
Regular FMAP Rate		Prior Year FMAP Rate[a]	Difference in FMAP Rate	Disaster-Recovery Adjustment Increase	Disaster-Recovery Adjusted FMAP Rate
	A	B	C = B - A	D = 50% × C	E = A + D
FY2011[b]	63.61	72.47	8.86	4.43	68.04
Second and Subsequent Years of Disaster-Recovery Adjustment Prior to P.L. 112-96					
Regular FMAP Rate		Prior Year Disaster-Recovery Adjusted FMAP Rate	Difference in FMAP Rate	Disaster-Recovery Adjustment Increase	Disaster-Recovery Adjusted FMAP Rate
	A	B	C = B - A	D = 25% × C	E = B + D
FY2012	61.09	68.04	6.95	1.74	69.78
Special Formula for FY2013					
Regular FMAP Rate		Prior Year Disaster-Recovery Adjusted FMAP Rate	Difference in FMAP Rate	Disaster-Recovery Adjustment Increase	Disaster-Recovery Adjusted FMAP Rate

Table 3. (Continued)

First Year of Disaster-Recovery Adjustment					
Regular FMAP Rate		Prior Year FMAP Rate[a]	Difference in FMAP Rate	Disaster-Recovery Adjustment Increase	Disaster-Recovery Adjusted FMAP Rate
	A	B	C = B – A	D = 50% × C[c]	E = A + D[d]
FY2013	61.24	69.78	8.54	4.27	65.51
Second and Subsequent Years of Disaster-Recovery Adjustment After to P.L. 112-96					
	Regular FMAP Rate	Prior Year Disaster-Recovery Adjusted FMAP Rate	Difference in FMAP Rate	Disaster-Recovery Adjustment Increase	Disaster-Recovery Adjusted FMAP Rate
	A	B	C = B - A	D = 25% × C	E = A + D[d]
FY2014	60.98	65.51	4.53	1.13	62.11

Source: Office of the Secretary, Department of Health and Human Services, "Adjustments for Disaster-Recovery States to the Fourth Quarter of Fiscal Year 2011 and Fiscal Year 2012 Federal Medical Assistance Percentage (FMAP) Rates for Federal Matching Shares for Medicaid and Title IV–E Foster Care, Adoption Assistance and Guardianship Assistance Programs," 75 *Federal Register* 80501; December 22, 2010. Office of the Secretary, Department of Health and Human Services, "Federal Financial Participation in State Assistance Expenditures; Federal Matching Shares for Medicaid, the Children's Health Insurance Program, and Aid to Needy Aged, Blind, or Disabled Persons for October 1, 2012 Through September 30, 2013," 76 *Federal Register* 74061, November 30, 2011; Office of the Secretary, Department of Health and Human Services, "Federal Financial Participation in State Assistance Expenditures; Federal Matching Shares for Medicaid, the Children's Health Insurance Program, and Aid to Needy Aged, Blind, or Disabled Persons for October 1, 2013 Through September 30, 2014," 77 *Federal Register 71420*, November 30, 2012.

[a] For FY2011, the preceding fiscal year's regular FMAP rate includes the application of the "hold harmless" provision under the ARRA temporary FMAP rate increase.

[b] Initially, the disaster-recovery FMAP adjustment was to go into effective on January 1, 2011. However, due to the extension of the ARRA FMAP adjustments, which extended the recession adjustment period to June 30, 2011 (the end of the third quarter of FY2011), no state qualified for the disaster-recovery adjustment until the fourth quarter of FY2011.

[c] The Moving Ahead for Progress in the 21st Century Act (MAP-21, P.L. 112-141) amended the disaster-related adjusted FMAP formula for FY2013 by changing the adjustment factor from a 25% to a 50%.

[d] The Middle Class Tax Relief and Job Creation Act of 2012 (P.L. 112-96) revised the disaster-recovery adjustment formula so that for the second and subsequent years the increase will be applied to the regular FMAP for that year rather than the prior year's disaster-recovery adjusted FMAP rate. Originally, this change had an effective date of October 1, 2013, but the Moving Ahead for Progress in the 21st Century Act (MAP-21, P.L. 112-141) changed the effective date to October 1, 2012.

In the fourth quarter of FY2011, Louisiana met the Stafford Act criteria (due to Hurricane Katrina and Hurricane Gustav),[31] and its regular FY2011 FMAP rate (63.61%) was at least three percentage points less than its regular FY2010 FMAP rate plus hold harmless from the American Recovery and Reinvestment Act of 2009 (P.L. 111-5) temporary FMAP rate increase (72.47%). As shown in *Table 3*, Louisiana's regular FMAP rate was adjusted 4.43 percentage points for a total FMAP rate of 68.04% for the fourth quarter of FY2011.

For FY2012, Louisiana met the Stafford Act criteria (due to Hurricane Katrina and Hurricane Gustav), and its regular FY2012 FMAP rate (61.09%) is at least three percentage points less than its FY2011 disaster-recovery adjusted FMAP rate (68.04%). As shown in *Table 3*, Louisiana's FY2012 disaster-recovery FMAP adjustment is 3.48 percentage points, which was applied to the FY2011 disaster-recovery adjusted FMAP rate for a total FMAP rate of 69.78%.

For FY2013, Louisiana meets the Stafford Act criteria (due to Hurricane Gustav), and Louisiana's regular FMAP rate for FY2013 (61.24%) is more than three percentage points lower than Louisiana's disaster-recovery adjusted FMAP rate for FY2012 (69.78%). As shown in *Table 3*, Louisiana's FY2013 regular FMAP rate is increased by 4.27 percentage points for a total FMAP rate of 65.51%.

For FY2014, Louisiana will meet the Stafford Act criteria (due to Hurricane Gustav), and Louisiana's regular FMAP rate for FY2014 (60.98%) is more than three percentage points lower than Louisiana's disaster-recovery adjusted FMAP rate for FY2012 (65.51%). As shown in *Table 3*, Louisiana's FY2014 regular FMAP rate will be increased by 1.13 percentage points for a total FMAP rate of 62.11%.

Conclusion

The FMAP rate is used to reimburse states for the federal share of most Medicaid expenditures. In FY2014, 15 states will have the statutory minimum FMAP rate of 50%, and Mississippi will have the highest FMAP rate of 73.05%. From FY2013 to FY2014, the regular FMAP rates for 36 states will change, while the regular FMAP rates for the remaining 15 states (including the District of Columbia) will remain the same.

Exceptions to the regular FMAP rate have been made for certain states, situations, populations, providers, and services. The ACA added a number of exceptions to the FMAP for "newly eligible" individuals, "expansion states," disaster-affected states, primary care payment rate increases, specified preventive services and immunizations, smoking cessation services for pregnant women, specified home and community-based services, health home services for certain people with chronic conditions, home and community-based attendant services and supports, and state balancing incentive payments.

Since federal Medicaid expenditures are a large and growing portion of the federal budget, controlling federal Medicaid spending has been a focus of federal deficit reduction proposals. Amending the FMAP structure has been identified as a way to reduce federal Medicaid spending by reducing the statutory FMAP floor.

Appendix. Regular FMAP Rates for Medicaid, by State

Table A-1 shows regular FY2006-FY2014 FMAP rates calculated according to the formula described in the text of the report (see "How FMAP Rates Are Calculated"). In FY2014, FMAP rates range from 50% (15 states) to 73% (Mississippi). From FY2013 to FY2014, regular FMAP rates will decrease for 22 states,[32] increase for 14 states,[33] and remain the same for 14 states[34] and the District of Columbia. All of the 14 states for which the FMAP rates do not change have the statutory minimum FMAP rate of 50%, and the FMAP rate for the District of Columbia is statutorily set at 70%.

Table A-1. Regular FMAP Rates, by State, FY2006-FY2014

State	FY06	FY07	FY08	FY09a	FY10a	FY11a	FY12	FY13	FY14	Change FY13 to FY14
Alabama	69.51	68.85	67.62	67.98	68.01	68.54	68.62	68.53	68.12	-0.41
Alaska	57.58	57.58	52.48	50.53	51.43	50.00	50.00	50.00	50.00	0.00
Arizona	66.98	66.47	66.20	65.77	65.75	65.85	67.30	65.68	67.23	1.55
Arkansas	73.77	73.37	72.94	72.81	72.78	71.37	70.71	70.17	70.10	-0.07
California	50.00	50.00	50.00	50.00	50.00	50.00	50.00	50.00	50.00	0.00
Colorado	50.00	50.00	50.00	50.00	50.00	50.00	50.00	50.00	50.00	0.00
Connecticut	50.00	50.00	50.00	50.00	50.00	50.00	50.00	50.00	50.00	0.00
Delaware	50.09	50.00	50.00	50.00	50.21	53.15	54.17	55.67	55.31	-0.36
District of Columbiab	70.00	70.00	70.00	70.00	70.00	70.00	70.00	70.00	70.00	0.00
Florida	58.89	58.76	56.83	55.40	54.98	55.45	56.04	58.08	58.79	0.71
Georgia	60.60	61.97	63.10	64.49	65.10	65.33	66.16	65.56	65.93	0.37
Hawaii	58.81	57.55	56.50	55.11	54.24	51.79	50.48	51.86	51.85	-0.01
Idaho	69.91	70.36	69.87	69.77	69.40	68.85	70.23	71.00	71.64	0.64
Illinois	50.00	50.00	50.00	50.32	50.17	50.20	50.00	50.00	50.00	0.00
Indiana	62.98	62.61	62.69	64.26	65.93	66.52	66.96	67.16	66.92	-0.24
Iowa	63.61	61.98	61.73	62.62	63.51	62.63	60.71	59.59	57.93	-1.66
Kansas	60.41	60.25	59.43	60.08	60.38	59.05	56.91	56.51	56.91	0.40
Kentucky	69.26	69.58	69.78	70.13	70.96	71.49	71.18	70.55	69.83	-0.72
Louisiana	69.79	69.69	72.47	71.31	67.61	63.61c	61.09c	61.24c	60.98c	-0.26
Maine	62.90	63.27	63.31	64.41	64.99	63.80	63.27	62.57	61.55	-1.02
Maryland	50.00	50.00	50.00	50.00	50.00	50.00	50.00	50.00	50.00	0.00
Massachusetts	50.00	50.00	50.00	50.00	50.00	50.00	50.00	50.00	50.00	0.00
Michigan	56.59	56.38	58.10	60.27	63.19	65.79	66.14	66.39	66.32	-0.07
Minnesota	50.00	50.00	50.00	50.00	50.00	50.00	50.00	50.00	50.00	0.00
Mississippi	76.00	75.89	76.29	75.84	75.67	74.73	74.18	73.43	73.05	-0.38
Missouri	61.93	61.60	62.42	63.19	64.51	63.29	63.45	61.37	62.03	0.66
Montana	70.54	69.11	68.53	68.04	67.42	66.81	66.11	66.00	66.33	0.33
Nebraska	59.68	57.93	58.02	59.54	60.56	58.44	56.64	55.76	54.74	-1.02
Nevada	54.76	53.93	52.64	50.00	50.16	51.61	56.20	59.74	63.10	3.36
New Hampshire	50.00	50.00	50.00	50.00	50.00	50.00	50.00	50.00	50.00	0.00
New Jersey	50.00	50.00	50.00	50.00	50.00	50.00	50.00	50.00	50.00	0.00
New Mexico	71.15	71.93	71.04	70.88	71.35	69.78	69.36	69.07	69.20	0.13
New York	50.00	50.00	50.00	50.00	50.00	50.00	50.00	50.00	50.00	0.00
North Carolina	63.49	64.52	64.05	64.60	65.13	64.71	65.28	65.51	65.78	0.27
North Dakota	65.85	64.72	63.75	63.15	63.01	60.35	55.40	52.27	50.00	-2.27
Ohio	59.88	59.66	60.79	62.14	63.42	63.69	64.15	63.58	63.02	-0.56
Oklahoma	67.91	68.14	67.10	65.90	64.43	64.94	63.88	64.00	64.02	0.02
Oregon	61.57	61.07	60.86	62.45	62.74	62.85	62.91	62.44	63.14	0.70
Pennsylvania	55.05	54.39	54.08	54.52	54.81	55.64	55.07	54.28	53.52	-0.76
Rhode Island	54.45	52.35	52.51	52.59	52.63	52.97	52.12	51.26	50.11	-1.15

Table A-1. (Continued)

State	FY06	FY07	FY08	FY09a	FY10a	FY11a	FY12	FY13	FY14	Change FY13 to FY14
South Carolina	69.32	69.54	69.79	70.07	70.32	70.04	70.24	70.43	70.57	0.14
South Dakota	65.07	62.92	60.03	62.55	62.72	61.25	59.13	56.19	53.54	-2.65
Tennessee	63.99	63.65	63.71	64.28	65.57	65.85	66.36	66.13	65.29	-0.84
Texas	60.66	60.78	60.56d	59.44	58.73	60.56	58.22	59.30	58.69	-0.61
Utah	70.76	70.14	71.63	70.71	71.68	71.13	70.99	69.61	70.34	0.73
Vermont	58.49	58.93	59.03	59.45	58.73	58.71	57.58	56.04	55.11	-0.93
Virginia	50.00	50.00	50.00	50.00	50.00	50.00	50.00	50.00	50.00	0.00
Washington	50.00	50.12	51.52	50.94	50.12	50.00	50.00	50.00	50.00	0.00
West Virginia	72.99	72.82	74.25	73.73	74.04	73.24	72.62	72.04	71.09	-0.95
Wisconsin	57.65	57.47	57.62	59.38	60.21	60.16	60.53	59.74	59.06	-0.68
Wyoming	54.23	52.91	50.00	50.00	50.00	50.00	50.00	50.00	50.00	0.00
Number with increase from previous year	9	11	18	21	25	17	16	12	14	
Number stayed the same from previous year	14	13	13	13	12	12	14	15	15	
Number with decrease from previous year	28	27	20	17	14	22	21	24	22	

Source: Department of Health and Human Services, Annual Federal Register Notices.

Notes: Reflects FMAP rates calculated using the regular FMAP formula, with exceptions noted below.

[a] FY2009-FY2011 FMAP rates do not reflect temporary increases provided under the American Recovery and Reinvestment Act of 2009 (P.L. 111-5) as amended by P.L. 111-226. In total, states received the temporary FMAP increase ran for 11 quarters, from the first quarter of FY2009 through the third quarter of FY2011 (i.e., October 2008 through June 2011).

[b] Section 4725(b) of the Balanced Budget Act of 1997 amended section 1905(b) to provide that the FMAP rate for the District of Columbia shall be set at 70% for purposes of titles XIX and XXI and for capitation payments and DSH allotments under those titles. For other purposes, the percentage for the District of Columbia is 50%, unless otherwise specified by law.

[c] Louisiana's FMAP rate was higher than the regular FMAP rate for this year due to the disaster-recovery FMAP adjustment. Louisiana's adjusted FMAP rate was 68.04% for the fourth quarter of FY2011, 69.78% for FY2012, 65.51% for FY2013, and 62.11% for FY2014. The disaster-recovery FMAP adjustment is discussed in the text.

[d] This FY2008 value of 60.56% was provided by HHS implementation of a DRA provision related to Hurricane Katrina. Using the regular FMAP formula, the state's FY2008 value would have been 60.53%.

End Notes

[1] For more information about the Medicaid program, see CRS Report RL33202, Medicaid: A Primer, by Elicia J. Herz.

[2] The Patient Protection and Affordable Care Act (ACA, P.L. 111-148 as amended) establishes 133% of federal poverty level (FPL) based on modified adjusted gross income (MAGI) as the new mandatory minimum Medicaid income eligibility level starting in 2014. On June 28, 2012, the United States Supreme Court issued its decision in National Federation of Independent Business (NFIB) v. Sebelius finding that the federal government cannot terminate the federal Medicaid funding a state receives for its current Medicaid program if a state refuses to implement the ACA Medicaid expansion. If a state accepts the new ACA Medicaid expansion funds, it must abide by the new expansion coverage rules. However, based on the Court's opinion, it appears that a state can refuse to participate in the ACA Medicaid expansion without losing any of its current federal Medicaid matching funds.

[3] For a broader overview of financing issues, see CRS Report R42640, Medicaid Financing and Expenditures, by Alison Mitchell.

[4] More detail about the exceptions to the regular FMAP rate is provided under the heading "FMAP Exceptions".

[5] For more information about CHIP, see CRS Report R40444, State Children's Health Insurance Program (CHIP): A Brief Overview, by Elicia J. Herz and Evelyne P. Baumrucker.

[6] Section 1905(b) of the Social Security Act.

[7] For example, assume that U.S. per capita income is $40,000. In state A with an above-average per capita income of $42,000, the FMAP formula produces an FMAP rate of 50.39%; if the formula did not include a squaring of per capita income, it would instead produce a higher FMAP rate of 52.75%. In state B with a below-average per capita income of $38,000, the FMAP formula produces an FMAP rate of 59.39%; if the formula did not include a squaring of per capita income, it would instead produce a lower FMAP rate of 57.25%.

[8] Preliminary estimates of state per capita personal income for the latest available calendar year—as well as revised estimates for the two preceding calendar years—are released in April. Revised estimates for all three years are released in September.

[9] Employer and employee contributions for government social insurance (e.g., Social Security, Medicare, unemployment insurance) are excluded from personal income, and earnings are counted based on residency (i.e., for individuals who live in one state and work in another, their income is counted in the state where they reside).

[10] Department of Health and Human Services, "Federal Financial Participation in State Assistance Expenditures; Federal Matching Shares for Medicaid, the Children's Health Insurance Program, and Aid to Needy Aged, Blind, or Disabled Persons for October 1, 2013 Through September 30, 2014," 77 Federal Register 71420, November 30, 2012.

[11] All the states with no change to their regular FMAP rates from FY2012 to FY2013 receive the statutory minimum FMAP rate of 50%, and the regular FMAP rate for the District of Columbia is statutorily set at 70%.

[12] Historically, Medicaid eligibility was generally limited to low-income children, pregnant women, parents of dependent children, the elderly, and people with disabilities. For more information about the ACA changes to Medicaid, see CRS Report R41210, Medicaid and the State Children's Health Insurance Program (CHIP) Provisions in ACA: Summary and Timeline, by Evelyne P. Baumrucker et al. When determining Medicaid eligibility for this group (and others) beginning in CY2014, states will be required to disregard a dollar amount of income equal to 5% FPL. The disregard will allow individuals at or below 138% FPL to enroll in the new eligibility group by reducing their countable income to 133% FPL or less.

[13] 132 S. Ct. 2566 (2012).

[14] For a discussion of the Supreme Court's decision on the Medicaid expansion, see CRS Report R42367, Medicaid and Federal Grant Conditions After NFIB v. Sebelius: Constitutional Issues and Analysis, by Kenneth R. Thomas.

[15] Congressional Budget Office, Estimates for the Insurance Coverage Provisions of the Affordable Care Act Updated for the Recent Supreme Court Decision, July 2012.

[16] In general, benchmark benefit packages may cover fewer benefits than traditional Medicaid, but there are some requirements, such as coverage of EPSDT services and transportation to and from medical providers, that might make them more generous than private insurance. For more information about benchmark coverage, see CRS Report R42478, Traditional Versus Benchmark Benefits Under Medicaid, by Elicia J. Herz.

[17] The "newly eligible" FMAP rates are available for these specific years, regardless of whether a state implements the ACA Medicaid expansion in 2014 or 2017.

[18] The coverage must include inpatient hospital services and cannot consist only of the following: premium assistance (or Medicaid coverage otherwise dependent on employer coverage or contribution), hospital-only plans, high-deductible health plans, or Health Opportunity Accounts under Section 1938 of the Social Security Act.

[19] However, by December 2009, the source notes that some (e.g., Maine, Pennsylvania, Washington) had closed enrollment in these programs. See Table 2 in Kaiser Commission on Medicaid and the Uninsured, Where are States Today?, December 2009.

[20] Expansion state FMAP formula = [regular FMAP + (newly eligible FMAP – regular FMAP) * transition percentage equal to 50% in CY2014, 60% in CY2015, 70% in CY2016, 80% in CY2017, 90% in CY2018, and 100% in CY2019+].

[21] Centers for Medicare & Medicaid Services, Frequently Asked Questions on Exchanges, Market Reforms and Medicaid, December 10, 2012.

[22] Currently, E-FMAP rates can range from 65% to a maximum of 85%. If the ACA increase applied in FY2011, nine states (Alabama, Arkansas, Idaho, Kentucky, Mississippi, New Mexico, South Carolina, Utah, West Virginia) and the District of Columbia would have a CHIP matching rate of 100%.

[23] Office of the Actuary, 2010 Actuarial Report on the Financial Outlook for Medicaid, Centers for Medicare and Medicaid Services, December 2010.

[24] Office of Management and Budget, Historical Tables: Budget of the U.S. Government, Fiscal Year 2012.

[25] Congressional Budget Office, Medicaid Spending and Enrollment Detail for CBO's March 2012 Baseline, March 13, 2012.

[26] Historically, Medicaid eligibility was generally limited to low-income children, pregnant women, parents of dependent children, the elderly, and people with disabilities; however, ACA requires Medicaid coverage for individuals under the age of 65 with income up to 133% of the federal poverty level. For more information about the ACA changes to

Medicaid, CRS Report R41210, Medicaid and the State Children's Health Insurance Program (CHIP) Provisions in ACA: Summary and Timeline, by Evelyne P. Baumrucker et al.

[27] Congressional Budget Office, An Update to the Budget and Economic Outlook: Fiscal Years 2012 to 2022, August 2012.

[28] CBO does not provide specifics about how far the FMAP floor would be lowered under their budget option. (Congressional Budget Office, Choices for Deficit Reduction, November 2012.)

[29] Initially, the disaster-recovery FMAP adjustment was supposed to be available beginning January 1, 2011. However, the disaster-recovery adjusted FMAP rate was not available until the fourth quarter of FY2011 due to the six month extension of the temporary FMAP rate increases provided through the American Recovery and Reinvestment Act of 2009 (P.L. 111-5) and extended by P.L. 111-226.

[30] To meet this criterion in the first year, a state's regular FMAP rate must have declined at least three percentage points relative to their regular FMAP rate from the preceding year. To meet this criterion in the second and subsequent years, a state's regular FMAP rate must have declined at least three percentage points relative to the preceding year's disaster-recovery adjusted FMAP rate.

[31] Hurricane Katrina was declared a major disaster under the Stafford Act on August 29, 2005, and Hurricane Gustav was declared a statewide disaster on September 2, 2008.

[32] The 22 states with regular FMAP rates decreasing from FY2013 to FY2014 are Alabama, Arkansas, Delaware, Hawaii, Indiana, Iowa, Kentucky, Louisiana, Maine, Michigan, Mississippi, Nebraska, North Dakota, Ohio, Pennsylvania, Rhode Island, South Dakota, Tennessee, Texas, Vermont, West Virginia, and Wisconsin.

[33] The 14 states with regular FMAP rates increasing from FY2013 to FY2014 are Arizona, Florida, Georgia, Idaho, Kansas, Missouri, Montana, Nevada, North Carolina, New Mexico, Oklahoma, Oregon, South Carolina, and Utah.

[34] The 14 states with regular FMAP rates remaining the same from FY2012 to FY2013 are Alaska, California, Colorado, Connecticut, Illinois, Maryland, Massachusetts, Minnesota, New Hampshire, New Jersey, New York, Virginia, Washington, and Wyoming.

INDEX

D

E

F

G

H

I

L

M

N

O